Essential Oils for Happy Living

MOTHER NATURE'S REMEDY
TO JUMPSTART HAPPINESS

Rebecca Linder Hintze

Visium Group LLC
LEESBURG, VIRGINIA

Portions of this book have previously appeared in *Living Healthy & Happily Ever After* and *Essentially Happy*.

This book is intended as a reference volume only, not as a medical manual. Its contents are not meant to diagnose or prescribe treatment for health conditions. The information contained is the idea of the author, based on research and life experience, and is not meant to replace professional medical treatment or substitute for the recommendations of your doctor. Please seek medical attention from a qualified medical professional when attempting to heal any physical or emotional condition.

Visium Group LLC
Leesburg, Virginia
www.rebeccahintze.com

Cover design by Nick Hintze
Author photographs by Katie Hintze, KNHPhoto.net

ISBN 978-0-9724297-8-8

Ordering Information:
Special discounts are available on quantity purchases by corporations, associations, and others. For details, contact the publisher at the website above.

Contents

I dedicate this book to you, my reader. These pages were put together with you in mind, and it is my wish and dream for you to live a healthy and happy life.

Foreword

I n this groundbreaking book, Rebecca Linder Hintze empowers us to look to ourselves, our thoughts, and our behaviors for personal and family healing. *Essential Oils for Happy Living* is the ultimate reference guide to parting the seas of your mind to gain a clear understanding of how powerful you are. Its holistic approach to healing is both refreshing and effective—however I am not surprised. As her husband, I have watched Rebecca work as a family issues expert and speaker on the topic of healing families for more nearly twenty years. Her ability to weed through the "junk" and pinpoint the root causes of the issues people present to her is remarkable. She has shared her gifts selflessly to help individuals and families unite and find peace and joy in life. Over these years, her several books have been translated in many languages and helped people all over the world to heal their households.

If you feel stuck in your efforts to get past something that's troubling you—whether it is physical or emotional—the combination of using the oil protocols in this book, understanding the greatness that already resides in you, and repeating positive affirmations on a daily basis will propel your conscious and unconscious mind into a state of peace, calm, and power.

Greatness is a label we put on people because of the accomplishments in their lives. But greatness is nothing more than people giving their best to whatever they set out to do. Greatness is innate in each of us, so you can trust that you are great just as you are. I encourage you to use this book to reach for and share your greatness, to become *bigger*. Love who you are, where you are, and what you are doing. Be humble and have gratitude for your life.

Essential Oils for Happy Living is more than an essential oils reference guide: It's a mindset and approach to life that's available to everyone. Happy living is not reserved for the few. It's not just a dream. By applying the concepts in this book, you will create positive change, changing yourself, your family, and all those with whom you share this mindset and approach to life for the better.

Every big movement in history started with the idea of one person. Though you may not change the world by putting essential oils on your feet and stating an affirmation, you'll change your own world. That's a good start!

—M. Shane Hintze

M. Shane Hintze worked for over twenty years in the telecommunications industry designing communication technology, including working with a team who created and launched the world's larg-

est satellite in space. Shane left his corporate vice president position in 2011 to support his wife in growing her essential oil business. Since that time, he's found tremendous joy and value working side by side with Rebecca while spending priceless time with their four children and two grandsons. The Hintzes have been married for more than twenty-eight years.

Definitions

It's quite possible that your healing process—or even the diagnostic process—would come to an immediate stand still the moment words like *neuropeptide, receptors,* and *neurotransmitter* were mentioned. *Whoa!* you think. *How am I supposed to get better if I can't even understand what we're talking about?*

Here's a quick look at some terms you'll come across as you read.

- *Neuron:* an impulse-conducting cell in the brain with specialized features that make it the functional unit of the nervous system. Up to 100 billion neurons are found in the human brain.
- *Neuropeptide:* a small protein-like molecule made from 3 to 40 amino acids that help neurons communicate with each other. Neuropeptides stimulate hundreds of activities in the brain and body, including food intake, learning, taste, smell, and memory.
- *Receptor:* a cell, usually a neuron, which receives stimuli from neuropeptides.
- *Neurotransmitter:* a substance that carries a nerve impulse, via a neuropeptide, from one neuron to another across a synapse.

Throughout this book, I often refer to affirmations—positive statements—that I suggest you use as you work with essential oils. Affirmations are powerful ways to support change in our lives.

When choosing an essential oil, I recommend researching the oil brand to ensure its oils are handled properly during production and are free from added chemicals and fillers.

Oils are best stored in dark, glass bottles to maintain their potency. Avoid oils stored in clear plastic bottles and—if you're shopping in a brick and mortar store—bottles covered in dust, which indicates they've been sitting around for a while.

Finally, steer clear of manufacturers who don't list the botanical name of an essential oil on their products or who sell all their oils for the same price. Essential oils that are the purest come directly from the plant and are priced according to the costs in production and availability of each type of plant. Some are more expensive.

Introduction

From the beginning of time, Mother Nature and human nature have coexisted, working with or against each other to create or destroy life, improve or diminish health. Most living things—human, animal, and plant—have proven adaptable to this process. If, for example, the soil changes or becomes depleted of the nutrients needed to keep a plant alive, a plant will shoot its roots deeper and wider below the surface to find the minerals and elements it needs to survive. We have the same instincts. Our desire to move consistently and continually forward, seeking to feel good—or just feel better—has led to the discovery of a wealth of knowledge and health in modern times. As human beings, we have figured out what makes us feel good and have moved in that direction for thousands of years.

Indeed, modern science and medicine can do more good for more people than our early ancestors probably ever dreamed. But sometimes, humanity's creations—which almost always point unfalteringly to the future—can impede our ability to look to the past and learn how our ancestors really lived and how they worked together with nature (instead of synthetics) to create happy and healthy lives. As the Chinese philosopher Confucius taught, "Study the past if thou wouldst divine the future."

Essential Oils and Emotions for Happy Living draws on both the past (meaning our roots with nature) and cutting-edge modern knowledge to deliver the science behind some of our ancestors' tried-and-true methods of finding health and happiness. In these pages, you'll discover how your own perceptions affect your mood, behavior, and health. You'll also find a wealth of detailed information about the use of plant science in treating both physical and mental ailments. Mother Nature has provided us with tools to help shift our perceptions—psychologically and emotionally—to jumpstart the healing process. *Essential Oils and Emotions for Happy Living* seeks to teach you how proper nutritional support— including vitamin supplementation, a healthy diet, exercise, drinking plenty of water, and using high-quality essential oils (the essence of plants)—can change your life!

The art of plant medicine has been practiced for thousands of years with much success according to anecdotal evidence. Today, medical science has begun documenting exactly how depression and other mental health disorders can be improved or resolved with a change of diet and exercise (Blumenthal et al., 2007). Well-respected doctors and researchers have also begun studying and promoting the effects of essential oils on infections, depression, and other ailments (Sarrell et al., 2003; Cappello et al, 2007; Fuchs, et al. 2005). The use of essential oils not only supports cellular communication and oxygenation, it also improves our neurochemistry by clearing receptor sites in the brain—which can alter our perceptions—and by supporting the production of neurotransmitters that make us feel happy.

During the years, I have worked with essential oils as a life coach and experienced surprising and wonderful results for my clients. Essential oils have helped individuals seeking all kinds of relief— resolving issues from lower back pain to depressed mood. A combination of oils, positive thinking, and deliberate application, seems to relieve the body of toxins, clear cell receptor sites, and create synergistic results unique to each person. Emotional healing has been both immediate and long term.

If you're like many others, you may be stuck in your process of trying to "feel good." You may have tried prescription drugs, therapy, or other wellness methods and yet plateaued in your journey to feel better. You may be suffering from learned behaviors that are limiting your good feelings and leaving you with patterns of self-defeat. You may be discouraged and depressed because you believe you've exhausted all possible means of improving your emotional state of being. The chapters of this book are meant to give you hope and to help you find natural and successful ways to move forward. We hope to provide the necessary tools to reestablish feelings of joy and happiness by natural means, thus making the relationship between human nature and Mother Nature one that works hand in hand toward progression and wellness.

Throughout the main text of the book, you'll find many oil protocols for typical mood and health ailments. Each protocol suggests a combination of essential oils—as well as a recommended application and a positive statement of affirmation—you can try as you experiment with this new process of feeling better. Additional protocols and helpful information about dozens of essential oils and oil blends can be found in an appendix, "Essential Oils Index" at the back of the book.

CHAPTER ONE

Your Thoughts as Chemical Reactions

U nderstanding the power of thought is the key to creating a healthy and happy life. Everything you perceive in the physical world has its origin in the invisible, inner world of your thoughts and beliefs. To become the master of your destiny, you must learn to manage the nature of your dominant, habitual thoughts. By doing so, you will be able to attract into your life that which you intend to create.

Albert Einstein said, "The whole of science is nothing more than a refinement of everyday thinking." Is it possible that Albert Einstein knew what modern science has shown us today: that our thoughts are physical—releasing chemicals inside our bodies the moment we think them?

The instant a thought occurs, your hypothalamus—the "control center" at the base of the brain—turns that thought into hundreds of neuropeptides, each associated with the dominant emotion of the corresponding thought. Those neuropeptides—your thoughts! —are actual molecules being transmitted through your mind and body. Candace Pert, Ph.D., world-renowned neuroscientist and pharmacologist known for pioneering much of the early work in mind-body medicine, discovered neuropeptides and found that they are carried through the bloodstream and transmitted from one neuron to another. Each neuropeptide interlocks with a special receptor on the receiving neuron's membrane, just like a lock fitting into a keyhole. The amino acids in each neuropeptide are then absorbed by your cells. In this way, your thoughts become a part of your body! And those cells can change depending on the nature of your thinking.

To Promote Clarity of Mind

Oil Protocol: Blend 4 drops frankincense, 3 drops Roman chamomile, and 2 drops wild orange.

Application: Use in a spritzer bottle to spritz the air around you and apply to the back of the neck, breathe deeply; put in a capsule and ingest; or apply directly to the throat and neck area in an upward motion.

Affirmations: I trust that I can hear and understand my innermost thoughts clearly. I own my thoughts. I think positively. I enjoy initiating good feelings instead of reacting to old patterns. Everything works out smoothly for me.

According to Dr. Pert's research, the body's cells develop more and more specialized receptors for the neuropeptides to which they are most exposed. In fact, cells will even begin to crave these neuropeptides and ask the hypothalamus to produce them. Over time your cells wind up supporting a self-fulfilling emotional prophecy all brought about by the power of thought. You get what you think about, no matter if you want it. Understanding the power of thoughts, therefore, becomes critical to permanently solving psychological and physical conditions (Pert, 1995; Pert, 1997).

The Daily News

Let's compare the process of your thoughts forming chemical reactions to the process of a news agency that writes and distributes the daily news. Every day writers and editors produce articles based on their research and perceptions of the latest information available in our world. The articles are then published in a newspaper or on the Internet. Similarly, you have opportunity every day to write your own news (choose your own thoughts) based on your perceptions of the happenings in your world. This news (your thoughts) is published in the form of neuropeptides that get delivered to the cells within your body. Just as world news becomes the reality of the world we live in, so do your thoughts create your own reality, which can include your health and well-being.

Every day, every moment, your cells wait for more information—the latest news—and then respond accordingly. When day in and day out you write the same morning news (provide the same thoughts) to your body, you establish patterns or pathways (specifically neuropathways) that leave you chemically altered. This is how habitual thinking patterns are created, and these patterns create matching body chemistry. Until different news is presented to your body on a regular basis, your neuropathways will guide you back to your original messaging or thinking.

Looking at thoughts in this manner makes it easy to see how repetitive negative thinking can manifest itself in a weak or sick body: Negative thoughts can become costly to your health as they quickly break down the whole body and leave it vulnerable to disease. Positive thinking, on the other hand, generates cellular vitality. Negative thoughts shatter the nervous system. Thoughts that are fear based or anger fueled break down cells, leaving the entire cellular system out of balance. Positive thoughts, particularly thoughts of love and gratitude, alter chemistry in positive ways, increasing cellular immunity. Understanding your own body chemistry and making lifestyle adjustments is central to jumping personal healing. Just as families need to communicate well to function effectively, just as companies need to offer adequate interoffice communication to stay profitable, the body's cells must communicate well within the body for it to stay healthy and the mind to be fully competent. Adjusting your cellular communication—or in other words, changing your thought processes—strengthens the body's natural ability to heal itself is.

A great way to look at this process is to think about what happens to your body when you are stressed and how that stress increases with each negative thought you produce.

Here's a simple example: Sarah is a mom with two young kids. The kids keep her active all day, leaving precious little time to accomplish the necessary tasks of running her small, part-time business. The income Sarah generates is vital to her family's livelihood. As time disappears, Sarah worries more and more about how to accomplish her goals. To combat the time slipping away, she stays up later at night, making her more tired each day. When exhaustion kicks in and she can't make her three-year-old son's play date, she chastises herself. She starts to think negatively about the way she mothers. The cycle continues as she decides to spend the evening focusing on the kids instead of work, and then realizes she will pay for it later when she gets behind at work. This will lead to negative thoughts about her capabilities as a businesswoman.

Somewhere in all of this, the sleep deprivation will lead to increased headaches and susceptibility to colds, which will consume more of Sarah's time. If Sarah uses negative thoughts to scold herself for not meeting her goals, she will continue the cycle.

Sarah's case demonstrates what dozens of scientific studies have concluded: Stress can be a hindrance. Add in some negativity, and the list of ailments that can follow or worsen with stress is huge: high blood pressure, back pain, weakened immunity, mental health conditions, adrenal fatigue, sleep disorders, and much more. There is no telling how many physical conditions are affected by stress.

Of course, all stress isn't bad. In fact, your immune system may benefit from short spurts of stress. The type of short-term stress that invokes a fight-or-flight response can help increase T-cells, the very thing the body needs to build the immune system and fight infection. You can experience the positive results of stress when you're hurrying to meet a deadline or cramming for an important exam.

Long-term stress from emotional overload, on the other hand, is not good for us. It is destructive to the immune system and to personal relationships. Stress means more conflict. Conflict contributes to arguments—sometimes violence—and this, in turn, may result in relationship troubles. Relationship challenges typically produce more stress, which leads back into a vicious cycle that may have begun in the first place with negative thoughts.

The mind is, indeed, a delicate and flexible tool that responds readily to the thoughts impressed upon it. Reprogramming your patterns of thought—rewriting the morning news, to extend our metaphor—is a powerful way to begin healing the mind and, in turn, the body.

Rewrite the News with Positive Affirmations

Many are unaware of their thinking patterns. That's not surprising, since much of what we think and feel is generated from our subconscious—the part of our minds that generates thoughts, feelings, and emotions automatically and mostly without our awareness. Austrian neurologist and psychoanalyst Sigmund Freud solidified the definition of the unconscious mind in the eighteenth century when he found evidence that repressed emotions and feelings from past experiences, as well as automatic skills and reactions, could be generated without conscious training or awareness. Knowing that much of what we process in thought form stems from our unconscious minds raises the important question, "How am I to change my thoughts if I'm not aware of their origination and they seem to occur without my knowing?"

In recent years, using positive affirmations to guide an individual's thoughts and break out of habitual, unconscious thinking has become increasingly popular and tremendously effective. There are even programs in the marketplace that employ subliminal means to speak to the unconscious mind, helping individuals to repattern thoughts at their deepest levels. Forms of hypnosis, acupuncture, meditation, rapid eye movement therapies, emotional freedom techniques (tapping certain points on the body while making statements), body talk therapies, emotional processing, various forms of energy work, emotional release through massage, and craniosacral therapy are only some of the many newer techniques used to help people change their instincts of thought and belief.

But simply deciding and committing to rewriting your thoughts on your own can also be a powerful way to make changes to your body chemistry. This process is important, even critical, to helping you create a happy and healthy life. Because of this, I've included positive affirmations throughout the book, both within the chapters and in the appendices, to help you better understand exactly how to rewrite the daily news within your cells and begin to create a happier and more fulfilled life—both inside and outside your body. Repeat these affirmations often. It is best to start affirmations when you are beginning a specific goal and feeling determined to achieve a specific result, not when you are in a bad space of feeling angry.

In addition, follow these five steps to help increase positive thoughts:

1. *Stop all criticism.* When you think and speak judgmentally and critically, you instantly walk under the dark cloud of negativity. Your attitude is affected, and the next thing you know, you're feeling down and blue. Think of it this way: If you wouldn't say it to or think it about a little child, don't say it to, or think it about anyone else. Especially, don't say it to or think it about yourself! To relieve patterns of self-criticism, apply 1 drop bergamot and 1 drop black pepper to the tip of your nose and the back of your neck. Black pepper helps break up unloving thought patterns, while bergamot helps to reestablish a sense of individual worth.

2. *Love.* Falling in love with someone is a wonderful experience. You are happy, your body responds with excitement, and you find

joy. Let yourself fall in love with someone all over again, whether it's a family member, a spouse, a friend, or even yourself! Remember, loving yourself doesn't mean you're vain. Vanity results when you're afraid you are not enough. True self-acceptance and love leave us joyful throughout our lives. Apply geranium and lime to the outside of the throat to help the mind and body continue to express joy.

3. *Laugh.* Not long ago, I visited my mother in a rehabilitation center in Massachusetts. My mother was recovering from knee replacement surgery. As part of her recovery, she was following a doctor's advice to laugh. To test out her doctor's theory that laughter would bring on a positive, healthy mood, she began laughing for no reason at all. Quickly the whole family got the giggles, and within minutes the whole room was hysterical! Everyone felt better almost immediately!

4. *Serve.* Happiness comes naturally when our thoughts and actions are focused on others. Find ways to give to others, and in so doing, you'll find that the universal law of abundance will flow your way. The essential oils clove, frankincense, and wild orange can be applied regularly to support abundance and a desire to reach out and serve.

5. *PPM—Pause, Pray, and Meditate.* Finding private time to pause, pray, and meditate is essential to our well-being. When diffused, sandalwood and myrrh help the mind to focus and become free of negativity, allowing individuals to more effectively pause, pray, and meditate.

To Generate a Positive Attitude and Focus

Oil Protocol: Blend 4 drops each bergamot and lemon with 3 drops each of basil and geranium.

Application: Diffuse and breathe deeply or rub on the back of the neck and up the front of the throat from the sternum while focusing on the following affirmation at least 3 times a day.

Affirmation: I trust myself to make good decisions for me. I find that the goals I set are very achievable and I easily manage the outcome. I am more comfortable with succeeding each day.

One of the greatest gifts of the day for a newscaster is the opportunity to take all the information collected for a newscast and dump it in the garbage, knowing that tomorrow brings new news, an opportunity for a different story. Yesterday's news is now history, so it's no longer that important. Luckily, brain and body chemistry allow for similar possibilities. You are not stuck in your thinking unless you choose to be stuck.

A Quick Primer on Essential Oils

Fortunately, Mother Nature knows just how to help us out of sticky spots. When it seems impossible to make a shift in mindset, essential oils—gifts from Mother Nature—spark our inner awareness and wake us up to possibilities of powerful personal change, growth, positive thinking, and better health!

Let's look at frankincense for an example of how this works.

Remember the receptor sites located on the cells throughout your body? Just like any body part, receptor sites can attract "cling ons." Think of a cling-on as junk that ends up where you don't want it—like cholesterol in your arteries, or the sticky leftovers of a cinnamon roll on your fingers, or negative scenarios that play on repeat in your mind. These cling ons block receptor sites and make transmissions from cell to cell sluggish.

We know that cling-ons in the form of cholesterol can be broken down by diet changes, exercise, and prescription medicine. Sticky fingers can be washed clean with soap and water. Sadly, modern science (in the form of medication) has yet to find a driver or a delivery system that can penetrate cell walls—let alone the lymphatic system or the blood-brain barrier—and get rid of the negative cling ons on cell receptors.

One of the miracles of frankincense is that its unique chemistry allows and facilitates oxygen crossing the blood brain barrier, thus making it an amazing property for soothing neurological imbalances and eliminating pathogens (part of the cling ons blocking cell receptor sites) from the hard-to-get-to areas of the brain, spine, and lymphatic systems. Simply put, frankincense can penetrate cell walls in a healthy manner and eliminate pathogens, toxins, and viruses from areas of the human body that scientists previously believed were closed off.

To Stimulate the Mind and Improve Clarity

Oil Protocol: Blend 10 drops each geranium, lemon, and rosemary with 5 drops each of basil, clove, and coriander, and 4 drops of white fir in a glass bottle.

Application: Add 4 or 5 drops to a water diffuser and diffuse regularly.

Affirmation: I am constantly striving to maintain clarity of mind. I have positive thoughts that make me happy. I enjoy being me. My mind is active, my body is active, and I love being me.

So, when you're lacking clarity or feeling stuck in a rut of negative thought, a simple application of frankincense—mixed with a little wild orange and applied to the forearms or deeply inhaled—can create a chemical response from the millions of molecules that rush through the body, facilitating changes in thought patterns and clarity.

As you'll learn throughout the book and in depth in the appendices at the back of this book, each individual essential oil works naturally and uniquely to enhance body chemistry. Combined with one another, oils can soothe headaches, backaches, and stomachaches, calm nerves, improve sleep habits, and more.

Using essential oils is easy. To begin, open the bottle and inhale the fragrance; then open to Appendix II, find the oil in question, and examine its benefits.

Three effective applications of most oils include:

Aromatic Use. Dispense several drops in hands, rub together, and inhale; or use a commercial diffuser and breathe deeply throughout the day.

Topical Use. Apply a few drops of the essential oil directly on the skin. I most frequently suggest applying to the bottoms of the feet, where absorption into the body systems happens quickly and effectively.

Internal Use. Drip one or two drops under the tongue, or mix in a glass of water and drink. You can also put drops in an empty veggie capsule and just swallow. When using internally, be sure to a brand labeled as safe for internal consumption.

How Much to Use and How Often?

With high-quality essential oils, less is always more. Adults should try an initial application of three to four drops on each foot or on the site of pain or distress (for example, apply to the core of the body for digestive issues). Because they are natural and harmless, you can always add more in ten to fifteen minutes. Adults can also try ingesting a capsule of three to four drops and waiting ten minutes before adding more to allow relief to take place.

For chronic or serious virus recovery, use oils every three to four hours, applying to feet or ingesting, and continue for four to five days after symptoms totally leave. As you use the oils more often, you will develop an understanding of their effectiveness and trust yourself to experiment and keep you feeling good.

Many people report that they benefit best when consuming lots and lots of water to facilitate removal of the debris the oils free up. Deep breathing is also helpful, as it releases toxins from the lungs and stimulates activity in the lower lobes of the lungs. Use inhalers prepared with essential oils to increase energy and motivate the positive changes you have chosen to implement.

Coupled with the advice that follows in this book, the use of essential oils has the power to change how you think about yourself and your life. Try out one of the "recipes" in Appendix I or Appendix II, breathe deeply, and then delve into the rest of the book. Your thinking may never be the same again!

CHAPTER TWO

Perceptions and Beliefs Guide Biology

The great playwright Oscar Wilde wrote, "We are all in the gutter, but some of us are looking at the stars." What are you looking at? For each of us, our own perceptions—the things we look at and think about most— are our reality. And perception is primarily shaped by our belief systems, which are formed in our families of origin and in our experiences with our culture. Developmental biologist and author of *The Biology of Belief*, Bruce Lipton, Ph.D., believes that perception is the primary mechanism that controls biology.

"Understanding on a scientific level how cells respond to your thoughts and perceptions," he writes, "illuminates the path to personal empowerment" (p. xvi). Understanding the role beliefs play in forming perceptions, changing the perceptions that don't work, and then embracing the tools Mother Nature has given us to help with this process are three essential keys to living a healthy and happy life.

To Identify Personal Power

Oil Protocol: Blend 4 drops geranium, 3 drops melissa, 3 drops rosemary, and 2 drops cinnamon in a glass roller bottle.

Application: Apply to the back of the neck in an upward motion and around the core of the stomach, while focusing on the following affirmations.

Affirmations: I trust that I can hear and understand my innermost thoughts clearly. I own my thoughts. I think positively. I enjoy initiating good feelings instead of reacting to old patterns. Everything works out smoothly for me.

Understanding How Your Beliefs Form Reality

Some scientists say that each person's reality is the projection of his or her awareness in the waking state of consciousness. What does that mean? It means that what you believe is true—or at least it's real for you. Best-selling author Stephen R. Covey explained in *The Divine Center* that when a man opens his mouth to speak, he in essence describes himself—his perception. Your perception is your reality. And even though the world around each of us may be different than we think it is, we don't see the differences because what we believe is real for us.

Does that mean if you change what you believe, you can also change your reality? Of course, the answer is yes! It also means that fear-based beliefs have tremendous power to negatively influence what you experience day to day. Often, it's not until a person becomes consciously aware of underpinning fears (or blocks) that he is willing or able to transform the picture of what he sees and experiences day to day. All too often individuals miserably live out their fears without uncovering the limiting thoughts and beliefs that rest deep inside themselves. Then they get stuck, reliving the same unhappy experiences again and again. Limiting beliefs are habitually the culprits behind frustration, unhappiness, relationship struggles, and depression, and often the cause of addiction.

To Be Willing to See the Truth

Oil Protocol: Blend 4 drops lemon, 3 drops ylang ylang, and 2 drops basil.

Application: Apply to the bones behind the ears and on the back of the neck.

Affirmation: I am willing to see the truth. I see myself through loving eyes.

Uncovering the Truth:
The Mind-Body Experience

So, how do you discover your limiting beliefs? Self-exploration be-comes a most effective answer! To change what's going on in your outer world, you must first change what's going on in your inner world. All wounds heal from the inside out. That's true for couples and fami-lies and individuals. No matter who's responsible for what pain you've experienced in the past (or the pain you continue to feel in the pre-sent), you must look to yourself to heal effectively.

And perhaps more important, you must eliminate or heal your limiting beliefs. How? By uncovering the truth! Let's say that deep down a person—let's call him Sam—believes (or fears) he's worth-less or not as good as others. Maybe Sam was abandoned, rejected, or abused at some point and thus wound up fearing that he was worthless or inferior. Consequently, Sam finds himself fearing and experiencing abandonment repeatedly. But when he uncovers the truth—that it was another's actions, not his own, that caused his abandonment—he will find that he's worthwhile and valuable, no matter his weaknesses, challenges, or faults. It's a universal truth that all people have glory within. There's goodness in us all. We must each choose to believe that and actively work to change until we discover that glory.

To Connect to Your Divine Goodness

Oil Protocol: Blend 5 drops wild orange, 4 drops frankincense, and 2 drops each of clary sage, lavender, and peppermint.

Application: Diffuse; or apply to wrists, back of neck, heart, and bottoms of feet.

Affirmation: I trust the goodness within me. I am connected and I listen to my inner voice. I trust the process of life.

Like computers with complex processing systems, the body contains all the facets of an individual's perception. Your personal body computer may change daily as new information is put in and outdated information is replaced by new understanding. Alternatively, your personal body "computer" may rarely change: running and rerunning old data. If you make decisions about others and yourself and lock these perceptions into your body/mind computer (usually by repetition), your system begins to filter your experiences through the beliefs and feelings you have stored.

Let's look again at Sam. His mind/body was fed constant cues about being unworthy every time he was let down as a young child of delinquent parents. Over time, Sam began to see all circumstances through a tainted lens—even after he was no longer surrounded by people who treated him poorly or with reckless abandon—blocking out other views of reality that exist simultaneously.

Here's another, more visual example of this concept. When you buy a new car, you become instantly familiar with that new model and color. In fact, from that point on you notice cars like yours whenever you are driving. In the past, you may not have really paid attention to navy blue Honda Pilots. But now you seem to notice every single one on the road. Fast forward ten years or more down the road, and it's likely you're still noticing all the navy-blue Honda Pilots on the road, even if you sold yours.

So it also is with each of us in our lives. When we have experiences that lead us to make decisions about our lives or ourselves, we unconsciously go out into the world and notice all other experiences that validate what we believe to be true. Certainly, there were just as many red Honda Pilots driving around all those years, but somehow you noticed only the navy-blue ones.

This is also the way the brain processes emotions and experiences. When the brain decides about an experience or an emotion, it often holds on to that perception and will attempt to recreate similar circumstances or feelings to validate those beliefs. Someone like Sam may expect that everyone abandons those they love. He may not recognize that healthy relationships do exist. Abandonment—his navy-blue Honda Pilot—is all he sees. Even if he parks right next to a shiny red minivan every day at work.

But Sam doesn't have to be stuck in this rut. He can start to notice the other cars on the road, to recognize that other paths exist, and that many, many relationships can move forward without any fear of abandonment. All he needs to do is start feeding his body and mind new information and changing his perceptions. This is true for each of us. Through self-exploration, take some time to discover the truth behind your beliefs, to look at the reality you have created and see if that reality might be skewed by your own perceptions. If it is, start feeding your mind new information. Reshape your reality and, in turn, you can reshape your vitality.

As you continue reading this book, you'll learn an important step in the healing process, which is discovering the natural resources that can help you restore vitality, lift your mood, and heal your mind and body as you work toward change. This is really what this book is about! Throughout each chapter, note the protocols and essential oils that might assist you in your journey. Refer often to the appendices for more ideas and information. And remember that Mother Nature offers humanity's oldest remedies for the ailments of human nature.

To Accept Your Gifts and Talents

Oil Protocol: Blend 3 drops each cilantro, myrrh, white fir, and ylang ylang, with 2 drops wild orange.

Application: Rub together in hands and inhale while focusing on the following affirmations.

Affirmation: I am accepting my unique gifts and talents now. I receive compliments, and my goodness expands daily. I trust myself to grow in positive ways. Every day I am getting better and better.

CHAPTER THREE

Emotions and Depression

The most important decisions we make—the ones that rule our lives and determine the outcome of our personal stories—are generally emotion based. Coming to understand your emotions will make you better equipped to improve yourself and perform better in all aspects of life. It can also help stave off depression.

Depression occurs for many reasons. And if you have been diagnosed with clinical depression, it is best to continue seeking the advice of your doctor and/or therapist. But we also hope the ideas in this chapter and throughout this book may serve as a valuable supplement in your journey to wellness. If you have not been medically diagnosed, but suspect you may be depressed, or if you simply struggle with confusion over your emotions and sadness because of it, you may find that Mother Nature has just the answers for you. Either way, understanding your emotions and learning how to deal with and resolve conditions of depression, will enable you to better live a happy and fulfilled life.

To Lift and Calm Your Mood

Oil Protocol: Mix 3 drops each in a glass roller bottle: bergamot, black pepper, cypress, sandalwood, and ylang ylang. For those with a diagnosed liver dysfunction, create this blend: 7 drops wild orange, 5 drops rosemary, 4 drops helichrysum, 4 drops Roman chamomile, and 3 drops geranium.

Application: Roll a big X on the right side of the center of your body (over the liver) with the first blend. For those with a diagnosed liver condition, in addition to drawing the X with the first blend, draw a circle around the X with the second blend. Repeat this protocol twice a day and drink a lot of water!

Affirmation: I recognize what makes me feel better. I am able to understand and sort my feelings in positive and helpful ways. My emotions support me. My feelings support my best and highest good. I am safe to examine my feelings and put them in proper prospective. I express my feelings in constructive and positive ways. I am happy with my feelings.

What Is Your Emotional Intelligence?

Carl Gustav Jung, Ph.D., the distinguished psychologist whose work has influenced psychiatry, religion, and literature for more than seventy years, said, "Emotion is the chief source of all becoming conscious." Feelings are amazing and complex in nature. They are unique to our individual experiences. And yet, nearly every emotion is common to each person on Earth. Fear, anger, sadness, frustration, resentment, terror, love, joy, peace, forgiveness, gratitude, and happiness—we all experience these feelings on one level or another throughout our lives. The balance and depth of these emotions is critical to leading a happy and healthy life. And I propose—along with many others—that your emotional intelligence (EI) is as important—If not more so—than your IQ.

A person's EI is defined as the ability to identify, use, understand, and manage emotion. It encompasses the following five characteristics and abilities (Salovey, 1990):

1. *Self-awareness*: knowing your emotions, recognizing feelings as they occur, and discriminating between them.

2. *Self-regulation:* handling feelings so they are relevant to the current situation and reacting appropriately; essentially, this is mood management.

3. *Self-motivation:* using emotions to direct yourself toward a goal, despite self-doubt, inertia, and impulsiveness.

4. *Empathy:* recognizing feelings in others and tuning in to their verbal and nonverbal cues.

5. *Social skill:* managing relationships, such as handling interpersonal interaction, conflict resolution, and negotiations.

In a 1995 report on the current state of emotional literacy in the United States, psychologist Daniel Goleman, Ph.D., states: "In navigating our lives, it is our fears and envies, our rages and depressions, our worries and anxieties that steer us day to day. Even the most academically brilliant among us are vulnerable to being undone by unruly emotions. The price we pay for emotional illiteracy is in failed marriages and troubled families, in stunted social and work lives, in deteriorating physical health and mental anguish and, as a society, in tragedies such as killings."

Goleman says the best remedy for battling emotional shortcomings is preventive medicine. In other words, we need to place as much importance on teaching our children how to develop emotional skills as we do on teaching them academic skills.

But before any of us can help our children master their emotions, we must have our own healthy emotions. This means learning how to better understand our thoughts, feelings, and underlying intentions, as well as being emotionally balanced and knowing how to direct emotional energy in positive ways.

The poet William Blake, in his epic work *Jerusalem,* wrote:

In your own bosom you bear your heaven and earth,
And all you behold, though it appears without,
It is within, in your imagination . . .

Becoming aware of your emotions is vitally important because your emotions guide you to know yourself and who you really are within. Self-awareness also helps you avoid the dangerous fallacy of projecting your own emotions on others.

Many experts say there are essentially two emotions—love and fear—and all other feelings exist somewhere on the continuum between them. Love is what you are born with, and fear is a learned condition that individuals experience while living on earth. When a person chooses to love, positive emotions dominate her experience. Emotions such as gratitude, joy, peace, forgiveness, and so forth, can manifest even during hard times. When a person chooses to live in a state of fear, however, negative emotions reign. Anger, judgment, sadness, burden, betrayal, control, and so forth tend to take over, even when the situation warrants only mild discomfort.

Knowing what you're feeling and why—and knowing how to handle your feelings and channel them in positive ways—is the key to mastering your thoughts and thus changing your body chemistry.

Emotional awareness begins by simply deciding you want to understand yourself. As you do so, you will receive the blessing of becoming more accepting of yourself—who you are, what you like, and what you need. You're likely to find that you understand others and are more compassionate. You will also become more motivated to accomplish your goals, make better decisions, and become a better communicator. All of this will help you to build healthier and happier relationships, which in turn, come back around to support a happy life style and healthy living.

To Balance Mood Swings and Get Clarity

Oil Protocol: Blend 4 drops each of frankincense, lemon, and rosemary, 3 drops each of lavender and white fir, and 2 drops each of fennel and rose in a roller bottle.

Application: Roll on and rub between hands and inhale; apply to bottoms of feet and lower back 3 to 4 times a day while focusing on the following affirmation.

Affirmations: I am more balanced and healthy in all aspects of my world each day. I am willing to allow myself to be human and imperfect without chronic criticism. I joyfully declare what makes me happy and I take steps toward living joyfully each day.

Dealing with Depression

More than 17 million Americans are affected by depression each year. Nearly everyone feels depressed from time to time. And there are circumstances in life that create *situational depression*, such as death, loss of job, illness, and so on. Generally, this type of depression passes after a relatively short period of time.

Clinical depression, on the other hand, lingers—often lasting months or years. It interferes with daily life on all levels—work, parenting, relationships, sleep, school, appetite, and so on. Situational depression can often turn into clinical depression.

Symptoms of clinical depression, also called *major depression,* may include:

- Persistently sad or irritable mood.
- Pronounced changes in sleep, appetite, and energy.
- Difficulty thinking, concentrating, and remembering.
- Physical slowing or agitation.
- Lack of interest in or pleasure from activities that were once enjoyed.
- Feelings of guilt, worthlessness, hopelessness, and emptiness.
- Recurrent thoughts of death or suicide.
- Persistent physical symptoms that do not respond to treatment, such as headaches, digestive disorders, and chronic pain.

The National Alliance on Mental Illness recommends, "When several of [the] symptoms of depressive illness occur at the same time, last longer than two weeks and interfere with ordinary functioning, professional treatment is needed" (NAMI, 2009, p. 1).

Diagnosing and treating mental health conditions involves many variables and differs from person to person. For some, prescription drugs help. For others, combinations of therapies help. Some find help from therapists, while others use a combination of prescription drugs and/or a variety of modalities. Some individuals seek a more holistic approach through exercise and better eating. Regardless of any treatment plan, proper nutrition and the use of essential oils can be powerful and supportive.

The tools I suggest in this chapter can help any individual suffering from a bout of short-term or situational depression. They can also help someone suffering from clinical depression, but should never take the place of consulting with a licensed medical professional.

One thing to consider if you deal with depression: Today, we know that our modern diet may be responsible for many cases of diagnosed depression and other mental health disorders. Food allergies have the potential to upset hormone levels and other key chemicals in the brain, resulting in symptoms ranging from depression to schizophrenia. Food allergies can also create inflammation in the body, a common occurrence in depressed individuals. Even if food allergies are not primarily responsible for a mental health condition, they can certainly aggravate it.

Additionally, the fungus *Candida albicans* can be a substantial contributor to mental health issues. Candida is a microorganism in the yeast/fungi family that gives off high levels of neurotoxins. While it is somewhat normal to have small amounts of candida in the body, under certain circumstances candida invades the body and shows up in organs and tissues where it doesn't belong, like the liver and kidneys.

Once it becomes entrenched in the body, the yeast itself systematically shares certain chemicals that affect cellular function. The results can be serious and long lasting, ranging from various forms of disease, to cases of mood disorders, depression, and anxiety. In fact, depression is one of the top three symptoms of candida.

If you believe you have an overgrowth of candida, I recommend that you stop eating white sugar, flour, and dairy, and drink lots and lots of water, until your condition improves. In addition, following an oil protocol for eliminating candida, such as applying a combination of melaleuca, frankincense, oregano, and thyme oil, diluted with a carrier oil, several times a day to the bottom of your feet and other affected areas of skin can be used to attain wellness and possibly eliminate depression.

To Release Grief

Oil Protocol: Blend 25 drops bergamot, 15 drops Roman chamomile, 7 drops cypress, and 6 drops marjoram in a glass vial.

Application: Pour 5 to 7 drops of blend into a water diffuser or attach the whole mixture to the side of a waterless diffuser, such as an Aroma-Ace® Diffuser. Run your diffuser for 15 minutes per hour when home.

Affirmation: I understand that grief is natural and I am letting it flow through me as appropriate. I am focusing on a future of love and acceptance and I know that it is okay to feel my feelings.

Seven Tools to Combat Depression and Other Mental Health Disorders

Experiment with the following tools to improve your emotional state.

First, consider setting realistic, small goals. Overdoing it can cause stress, which only makes things worse. It's always good to reward yourself for even the smallest of accomplishments. When you focus on what you can and have accomplished, rather than on what you didn't or can't accomplish, you set yourself up to be both happier and healthier.

Second, find a support system to help lift the fog of depression. This may feel counterintuitive at first because depression makes its sufferers instinctively want to walk away from others, shut down, and hide. Resist the instinct to isolate yourself and reach out instead. This is an important part of the recovery process.

Third, exercise. Whenever you can and however you're able, move your body in a positive motion. If you're up to running, do it. If a brisk walk is better, try it. Swimming may be your thing, or yoga. In whichever way you can appropriately exercise, start doing it right away. But don't forget my first piece of advice: Set a realistic goal.

Regular exercise not only prepares us physically, mentally, and emotionally to function better in our relationships with others, it also helps us feel and look better! Doctors frequently recommend exercise for a variety of reasons, including both its physical and psychological benefits. There is great evidence today that exercise slows down the effects of aging and builds the body's defenses against disease and emotional stress. It also helps reduce the chance of breast cancer in women over the age of forty (McCullough, et al., 2012).

Fourth, be sure to sleep. Without a good night's sleep, the risk of developing a mood disorder goes straight up. Lack of sleep can be the root cause of a variety of mental health disorders. Sleep is essential to balancing brain chemistry, particularly melatonin and serotonin levels, which work synergistically to keep us feeling rested and happy. The body naturally produces melatonin after the sun goes down in the evening. Late use of electronics, where there's light behind a screen, slows down the body's natural production of melatonin. Because of this, those who struggle to sleep (really, anyone who wants to sleep well) should avoid viewing any form of electronics after 9 P.M.

According to the National Institutes of Health, "Sleep appears necessary for our nervous systems to work properly. Too little sleep leaves us drowsy and unable to concentrate the next day. It also leads to impaired memory and physical performance and reduced ability to carry out math calculations. If sleep deprivation continues, hallucinations and mood swings may develop. Some experts believe sleep gives neurons used while we are awake a chance to shut down and repair themselves. Without sleep, neurons may become so depleted in energy or so polluted with byproducts of normal cellular activities that they begin to malfunction. Sleep may also give the brain a chance to exercise important neuronal connections that might otherwise deteriorate from lack of activity" (2007).

To help you sleep at night, place lavender oil on your pillow or on the insides of your forearms and/or massage on your ear lobes. Essential oil blends that may help at bedtime include a grounding blend made of blue tansy, frankincense, rosewood, and spruce; vetiver mixed with any citrus oil; and a calming blend made of lavender, Roman chamomile, sandalwood, vanilla, and ylang ylang. Apply one of these blends on the throat, neck, ears, backs of knees, or the bottoms of the feet. For those who struggle with bad dreams, apply vetiver and myrrh across the top of the chest. If you're working with a child who is experiencing night terrors, try diffusing lavender, bergamot, or vetiver in the child's bedroom at night.

Fifth, drink more water. We all need to be drinking more water and less of the many other liquids we like to consume. The body is made up primarily of water; and the brain, especially, needs plenty of water to work correctly. It's a bit funny that we know our cars won't run without gas, but we often forget that our bodies won't run well without certain vital contributors—like nutrients from food and water.

Here's an example of how drinking water communicates health to every part of your body. Think about the last time you broke in a new pair of shoes and ended up with a big blister on the bottom of the foot. To compensate, did you adjust the way you moved your entire body to prevent pain from shooting out your foot? Did your whole leg start to ache after favoring the other one for hours? Were you grumpy by the time you took off your shoes at the end of the day? The body works the same way. If just one element is out of place, the whole body adjusts to make up for the difference. If that element is water— the element that makes up to 60 percent of our insides—you know there is going to be trouble. Hydrating the body aids in cell replacement, waste elimination, and brain functioning. If you are low on overall water intake, you're on your way to being more toxic, crabbier, more sluggish, and less capable of setting and achieving important goals.

Sixth, analyze your nutritional intake and then improve it. Our cells are like us: They need to eat, breath, eliminate, and rest daily to function well. Proper nutrition is fundamental to the body's ability—and even each individual cell's ability—to work correctly.

Take some time to look at what you eat. For years, we were told to avoid fat. The food industry helped us out by producing "low-fat," "lite," and "no-fat" versions of nearly every packaged food product available. When manufacturers removed the fat, other ingredients—namely, sugar—were added to make up for the loss in taste and texture. The additions often meant an increase in calories, so eating one serving of the low-fat version of a food could mean consuming more calories than one serving of the full-fat version. We were eating less fat, but gaining weight. And we were still hungry after eating more! Fat not only makes things taste better, it also leads to satiety—feeling full—and thus encourages us to stop eating sooner. Foods that are lower in fat, but higher in simple carbohydrates, like sugar, take less time to digest and are thus less filling.

If all that wasn't enough to make us eat more low-fat products, there was also the label itself telling us which food choices to make. A study conducted at Cornell University's Food and Brand lab found that consumers are likely to eat more of a product that is labeled "low-fat" than they would eat of the same product without such a label. In fact, study participants ate 28 percent more M&M candies if the candies were picked from a bowl with the label "new, low-fat M&Ms" (Wansink, 2006). Such a product does not actually exist, but plenty of other foods labeled "low-fat" do exist, and it's likely many of us eat more of those foods simply because of the label.

Not only has the low-fat fad led to eating more sugar, and more calories overall, it has also led to deficiencies of *good fats*. Let's look at polyunsaturated fat. Polyunsaturated fats are essential for several healthy, normal functions. They help build cell membranes and the protective sheaths around nerves. They play a vital role in blood clotting, muscle contraction, and control of inflammation. They improve cholesterol levels by reducing LDL (the bad form of cholesterol), and they help lower triglycerides. Polyunsaturated fats include omega-3 fatty acids and omega-6 fatty acids. Both omega-3 and omega-6 fatty acids have been shown to reduce the risk of heart disease. And omega-3 fatty acids have been shown to improve the risk of stroke and possibly provide benefits in the treatment of lupus, eczema, and rheumatoid arthritis.

We need to eat *more* of these good fats. Omega-3 fatty acids are abundant in fish, such as halibut, salmon, mackerel, and trout. But they can also be found in walnuts, flaxseed, Brussels sprouts, kale, watercress, and other green leafy vegetables.

Monounsaturated fats, when eaten in moderation and as a replacement for saturated and trans fats, are the other healthy fat. Monounsaturated fats help reduce levels of LDL in your cholesterol, which reduces the risk of heart disease and stroke. They also provide nutrients that enrich and maintain cell development, mainly vitamin E. Olive oil, peanut butter, avocados, macadamia nuts, almonds, and most other tree nuts are also good sources of monounsaturated fats.

So, if you're going to read labels, make it the label on the back of packaged food. If fat is listed, make sure it's the good kind. If the front of the label touts the item as being low fat, check out how much sugar is in the product. Stay away from products that list sugar as one of the first three or four ingredients. Better yet, buy whole foods that don't need to come with labels because they come from nature. The food that goes in your mouth impacts nearly every system in your body, from metabolism to bone density to muscle tissue to the circulatory system. When you decide to put something in your mouth, ask yourself if it is likely to improve these systems or damage them.

Seventh, regularly diffuse citrus oils. Our most powerful sense is the sense of smell. Scent imprints memory! The limbic system of the brain sits right behind the nasal cavity. Thus, aromatic use of essential oils, particularly citrus oils, becomes a powerful way to reach and impact brain function. Citrus oils are particularly amazing because they are fast and direct. They throw themselves on debris and clear the junk in our minds, all the while enabling healthy cells to do their jobs better. They literally increase neurotransmitter activity in the brain (making us feel happier and less stressed) and they eliminate pathogens, keeping us healthy and well! Citrus oil compounds are energizing and smart. They are fantastic cleaners inside our body systems and they improve mental clarity. (See, for example, Mayer, 2007.)

Citrus oils are remarkable at clearing receptor sites in the brain and reducing stress. Just a simple deep breath of any all-natural high-grade citrus oil may help reduce anxiety and bring almost instant thoughts of joy and peace. Bergamot, for example, is both a powerful citrus oil and a positive neurotonic—good for the brain. Really, any high-quality essential oil will serve the body in some way emotionally, offering instant relief and support.

To Relieve Emotional Trauma

Oil Protocol: Combine 4 drops each in a roller bottle: cilantro, coriander, frankincense, helichrysum, vetiver, white fir, and wild orange.

Application: Apply to lower back and outside of ankles in an upward motion.

Affirmation: I am allowed to be healthy. I heal rapidly and immediately. My body is whole and complete. I trust myself to take care of myself. I am rapidly recovering, and every day I create positive feelings I am comfortable with.

If you're depressed, watch those negative thoughts! And use your essential oils and the protocols listed throughout the book and the appendices to help you create new ways of thinking about yourself, your life, and your environment.

Perfectionism:
A One-Way Ticket to Negative Emotions

For perfectionists, life becomes a one-way ticket to unhappiness as negative emotions take over, potentially resulting in depression and addiction. A perfectionist is one who strives for flawlessness and high achievements. What gets a perfectionist into trouble is the desire to be perfect turning into a focus on avoiding failure. This negative focus drags perfectionists into an emotional puddle of misery. Trying to avoid failure is counterproductive in a world where we often learn best from the mistakes we make!

Perfectionists learn early in life to gain approval and love from others by accomplishing or achieving. Consequently, the self-esteem of a perfectionist is based primarily on external standards. This leaves a perfectionist vulnerable and sensitive to the opinions of the world around them. To protect themselves from criticism or ridicule, perfectionists work very hard to be perfect. Ultimately, this is how they perceive they get love. And since human beings are naturally most concerned about being loved (subconsciously we thirst after love as much as we desire food and water), a perfectionist works very hard, exhaustingly hard, to be all things to all people. Because gaining the approval of others doesn't bring us love and acceptance (self-approval must provide that need), a perfectionist can end up being miserable, processing all kinds of negative emotions like fear, sadness, guilt, shame, and even anger.

For perfectionists, the following show up regularly: fear of failure, fear of making mistakes, fear of disapproval, all-or-nothing thinking (which leads perfectionists to be out-of-balance and often lose prospective), an overemphasis on "shoulds," believing that others are easily successful (but not them), and a lot of guilt and judgment.

There is a healthy side to perfectionism, though. In fact, psychologists now group perfectionism into two categories, *adaptive* (healthy) and *maladaptive* (unhealthy). The difference: Healthy perfectionists aren't afraid of failure. They remain self-confident when high standards are set, even if they can't seem to keep up. A maladaptive (unhealthy) perfectionist lives in a world of self-beat-up, never feeling good enough and rarely feeling happy with her accomplishments.

Perfectionists typically don't know who they are. They are commonly lost to their own thoughts and feelings, always living in a world of "shoulds" that are initiated by the opinions of others. Perfectionists live with a lot of guilt, personal sabotage, and shame. They have little or no self-worth. When others provide any kind of feedback in their lives, they are never satisfied! They don't know how to feel personal satisfaction.

To break out of patterns of perfectionism and self-sabotage and let go of any "shoulds" that may have defined you, apply this "Should Away" Blend: combine 4 drops cilantro, 4 drops peppermint, 3 drops lavender, and 3 drops wild orange in a roller bottle. Apply behind the ears and on the back of the neck and focus on this statement: I am comfortable with choosing to feel good all the time.

Nobel Peace Prize winner Nelson Mandela writes: "In judging our progress as individuals, we tend to concentrate on external factors such as one's social position, influence and popularity, wealth and standard of education . . . but internal factors may be even more crucial in assessing one's development as a human being: honesty, sincerity, simplicity, humility, purity, generosity, absence of vanity, readiness to serve your fellow men—qualities within the reach of every human soul" (in Maharaj, 2006, p. 166).

Dealing with Anger

Ralph Waldo Emerson is reported to have quipped, "For every minute you are angry you lose sixty seconds of happiness." Each of us experiences anger. Fortunately, when anger is managed in healthy ways, it can be a good thing! Well-managed anger can be a catalyst for change and often motivates people to action. However, poorly managed anger, like any other poorly managed emotion, can become a raging fire with the power to burn down a house.

Unsurprisingly, anger usually has company. It is best friends with the emotions fear and sadness. In fact, we call anger a secondary emotion because the root of anger is found in other, deeper feelings.

To Diminish Anger

Oil Protocol: Blend 16 drops peppermint, 14 drops rosemary, 12 drops bergamot, and 4 drops white fir in a glass vial.

Application: Pour 5 to 7 drops of blend into a water diffuser or attach whole mixture to the side of a water diffuser.

Affirmation: I am learning to understand the root cause of my anger. I am making wise choices to sleep, heal, talk, and release my anger. I am happy with who I am. I am replacing anger with joy.

If you're dealing with anger, here are a few tips to try.

Understand your anger. It's always easier to deal with your emotions when you understand why you're really upset. When stress builds, or you are sleep deprived, starving, or sick, handling your emotional load becomes close to impossible. Losing your temper is often the *resulting* action. Figure out what led you to that action.

Learn to express your anger constructively. Talk with a trusted friend or therapist about your anger. Go to the basement or a closet and shout out your grievances. Write your thoughts in a journal. Coloring out your feelings—even your ugliest thoughts—with crayons on paper can be surprisingly helpful. You can always tear up or burn your writings or drawings once you've released them on paper.

Remember the word constructively *as you work to express your anger.* Overthinking and over-talking can add fuel to the fire. If you find yourself seeking evidence to support your negative state (talking to rant instead of talking to heal), you aren't doing yourself any good. Going over and over facts repeatedly adds to stress, potentially increasing the body's stress hormones (cortisol levels) and thus negatively impacting health. Women, especially, get involved in conversations that are basically complaint sessions that tend to travel in downward spirals. If you feel yourself heading in this direction, change the subject to a happy, healthier topic and consider finding a safe person who will support a productive conversation.

To Relieve Anger

Oil Protocol: Blend 3 drops each black pepper, geranium, melissa, and wild orange in a glass vial.

Application: Apply to the throat, sternum, and bottoms of the feet both morning and night.

Affirmation: I manage my emotions with ease and understanding. I am confident in my ability to remain calm and peaceful at all times.

Exercise. Yep! Here it is again. Exercise cures many ailments. Indeed, one of the best tools for managing anger is exercise. When you are terribly upset or angry, head to the treadmill, take a brisk walk, pop in an exercise video, take a jog or swim, or do a little yoga. This can help release pinned-up feelings inside your body and provide instant relief.

Our Responsibility to Be Happy

Your mood has a powerful effect on the world around you. Just think about it: How easy is it for one grumpy child (or parent) to ruin the environment of a home? Can one enraged, negative employee destroy the tone of an entire office? It's always true that one bad apple has the potential to ruin the entire barrel. That's why we each have a personal responsibility to choose happiness, not just for our own benefit, but also for the benefit of others.

During a study on meditation years ago, several doctors working with mind/body expert Deepak Chopra identified that serotonin levels in the brain increase during meditation. (Serotonin is a neurotransmitter involved in the transmission of nerve impulses in the brain; a steady level of serotonin helps individuals maintain a happy feeling, while lower levels of serotonin may result in mood disorders or sadness). After further exploration, the group of physicians realized that those who were not participating in the actual process of meditation, but were involved with the study on a regular basis also experienced an increase of serotonin in the brain. In other words, the study gave a profound indication that happy feelings spread. Positive attitudes create energy that physically impacts those with whom we associate on a regular basis.

Do you sometimes feel drained when you're in an environment with extraordinarily negative people? It's possible that what you're feeling may be more than just an emotional response; their negativity may be affecting you physically. Conversely, think of the benefit it is to you and others when you focus on the positive, seek out good in all you do, fill your mind with uplifting thoughts, and influence those around you with positive thought energy.

When we are selfish, we think only of our needs. Selfish people are generally very unhappy. But those who forget themselves in the service of others find happiness. When you feel grumpy, sad, or just plain miserable, remember your personal responsibility to be happy and begin to serve others by healing your grumpy mood. Fulfill your responsibility to be happy by turning your negative tone into a positive influence.

To Maintain Positive Energy Around You

Oil Protocol: Use a commercial blend intended to bring joy; or make your own by blending 2 drops each cypress, lavandin, lemon myrtle, melissa, sandalwood, tangerine, and ylang ylang.

Application: Apply behind the ears.

Affirmation: I am maintaining extraordinary positive energy and healthy boundaries. Everyone I encounter is happy, helpful, delightful, and supports me in multiplying positive energy in my environment.

That may seem easier said than done. And it is. When you are emotionally overloaded and can't muster up the ability to put a smile on your face, forcing an instant change of mood isn't realistic. So here are some tips for clearing the dark cloud and bringing in powerful light.

1. Apply a respiratory oil blend—such as a mix of eucalyptus, laurel leaf, lemon, peppermint, and tea tree (*Melaleuca*) oils—on your chest and visualize blowing all your frustrations, fears, anger, or whatever you're feeling into an imaginary balloon. Watch inside your mind as the balloon lifts high in the sky, eventually exploding in the light of the sun.

2. Diffuse white fir essential oil as you write out your negative feelings in a journal. When you're done, go over your thoughts and record all that you've learned from your negative experiences.

3. Diffuse or apply lemon essential oil while you listen to beautiful, uplifting music.

4. Apply peppermint essential oil and go for a walk out in nature.

5. As the character Maria in *The Sound of Music* (originally played by Julie Andrews) might suggest, make a list of your favorite things, and be sure to include all that you're grateful for. Pick three of the essential oils from the list below and apply on the forehead and temples before you begin writing down your favorites: clary sage, eucalyptus, rose, rosemary, white fir, and wild orange.

CHAPTER FOUR

The Family Connection

The late American screenwriter Frank Howard Clark once said, "Habit is something you can do without thinking, which is why most of us have so many of them." And where are most of these habits developed? In our families of origin. The families we come from do much to shape our behaviors, which is why it becomes important to look carefully at any negative behaviors picked up simply because we were born in a certain place or time.

For Healing Family Issues

Oil Protocol: Combine 4 drops each in a roller bottle of basil, bergamot, fennel, lemon, rosemary, and white fir.

Application: Roll on the left shoulder from front to back; apply two to three times a day when a destructive pattern emerges, stating the affirmations below while applying.

Affirmation: I am safe. I create a safe and loving world. I am loved. I love and accept myself. I am comfortable changing my perceptions. I am free to be me.

Many patterns of behavior learned in the home thrive for generations simply because no one in the family realizes there is any other way to do things. Some of these patterns may be destructive and damaging to individuals. Others may simply be less than effective. Consider this somewhat funny example of the latter: One day a newly married woman was getting ready to put a ham in the oven for her first Sunday dinner at home with her new husband and his family. Her husband watched with questioning eyes as she pulled the ham out of the refrigerator to prepare it and immediately cut off two inches from both ends. She glazed the ham, plopped it in the pan, moved it to the oven, and then unceremoniously threw away the ends of the ham! It took a little courage to question his new wife as she readied the rest of the meal, but the husband finally blurted out, "Why on earth did you throw away those perfectly good ends of the ham?"

Baffled, the wife responded, "Well, isn't that the way you're supposed to cook a ham?" After some discussion with her husband, the wife decided to call her mother to get proof that this, indeed, was the proper way to cook a ham. "Mom," she said, as she handed her husband the phone in exasperation, "will you please explain to Joe why it's important to cut off the ends of the ham." Her mom somewhat sheepishly replied that she didn't actually know the reason; she'd just watched her own mother prepare ham that way for years. This prompted a call to Grandma . . . and a good laugh a few weeks later after the proverbial smoke of the argument had cleared.

Grandma's response? "Well, I only had this tiny pan. The hams your grandfather brought home from the butcher never fit, so I just cut off the ends. Maybe I should have bought a bigger pan."

Take a moment and think about the story of the ham. The consequences of following precedent without question were small here. But what if the precedent isn't in how you cook a ham, but how you react to a child who shatters a plate or a spouse who doesn't do exactly what you ask. If you're the first in a family line to want to break an ineffective or unhealthy pattern, changing may seem more impossible than moving a mountain. But it's not. It takes time, work, and more time. But it is possible. And worth it.

How do you transform bad habits that have been ingrained for generations? Complete answers are found in detail in my book *Healing Your Family History* (2006). Those who work through my five-step process find great success transforming the habits that are blocking them from success! This chapter provides an overview of the process to get you started.

To Facilitate Powerful Change

Oil Protocol: Blend 4 drops helichrysum, 3 drops Roman chamomile, 3 drops sandalwood, and 2 drops lavender.

Application: Rub around your core and sternum.

Affirmation: I enthusiastically go with the flow. I joyfully embrace positive change in my life.

Where It All Begins

Certainly, we are vulnerable when we are born. Not only are our tiny, delicate bodies dependent on others for the basics of life—food, safety, and shelter—but we also look to our parents, family members, and even our culture for our sense of value and purpose. Early on, our parents, teachers, leaders, and communities play a huge role in dictating who we are and what we will become. Because we are young and impressionable in our early years, we tend to absorb verbal and non-verbal scripts—or patterns of thinking about ourselves—and we typically create our lives accordingly, unless (or until) we become enlightened otherwise.

Our perceptions of ourselves are often based on the opinions, thoughts, and comments of others. It's common that when a mother believes her child is bound for success and is beautiful and gracious, the child will tend to grow up to be successful, to radiate beauty and graciousness. To the contrary, if a parent projects that her child is a troublemaker, foolish, selfish, or worthless, it's likely the child will manifest the negative script and think and behave accordingly. Because our feelings about ourselves shape our lives, understanding these scripts (or the roles we're assigned by others) and their effects on us is crucial. And understanding and rewriting the unhealthy scripts we project on others is also crucial.

The good news is that you can rewrite your daily news by changing the scripts—not only the ones given to you, but the ones you give to others. You don't have to give your power away to the opinions of others, and you can teach your loved ones that they don't have to do it either. The great runner, author, and philosopher George Sheehan said, "Success means having the courage, the determination, and the will to become the person you believe you were meant to be."

So how do you change the scripts and help yourself think differently? First, you need to know what you want, who you really are, and what you desire to become. You need a vision of your highest and best self and you need a dream. And then you must be anchored in this purpose. Basil, bergamot, myrrh, patchouli, thyme, and vetiver are essential oils that support us in broadening our minds, changing our scripts, tearing down personal blocks, and helping us become who we want to be.

New York Times best-selling author Gregg Braden tells a powerful story in his book The Divine Matrix (2006). He explains how invincible we are when we fully focus ourselves on a meaningful dream. He said that years ago he was enrolled in a martial arts class. One day he showed up for class and the teacher announced a change in schedule.

The teacher told the group (some of his finest students) that he wanted them to knock him over. He took a minute to anchor himself to the ground. Assuming the task was easy, a few students tried to shove him. When they realized he wasn't budging, the whole group ganged up on one side to knock him over. Still, he remained stable and strong. Why?

Later the teacher explained that before the exercise, he had anchored himself deep within his consciousness by strongly visualizing that he was sitting between mountains and that he was chained to his position. His perceived reality became so strong that it outweighed the laws of physics. In other words, his dream (or vision) was so solid no one could topple it.

When your thoughts, beliefs, and chemistry support you in being solid in who you are, regardless of your family history, you become able to withstand the judgments, criticisms, attacks, and hurtful projections of others. Likewise, when you are solid in your dreams, you can overcome all odds and achieve them.

To Combat Fear

Oil Protocol: Blend 20 drops bergamot, 20 drops clary sage, 6 drops cypress, 6 drops ginger, and 4 drops fennel in a glass vial.

Application: Pour 5 to 7 drops of blend into a water diffuser or attach the whole mixture to the side of a waterless diffuser.

Affirmation: I am capable and strong. I feel joy daily. I am safe. I have enough and I am enough.

Costly Family Beliefs

All families pass along traditions. Some traditions promote success, encourage love, and serve and heal those who choose to participate. Others can be both negative and positive. Some family traditions come without any good. Families who pass along dark abuse and hate pass along traditions that must be eliminated for a family (even society) to heal and experience long-term joy, peace, and love. Most families don't intend to pass down destructive messages to their descendants. In fact, most parents want more for their children than they had for themselves.

Why should any of us take the time to identify our family beliefs or traditions? The reason is twofold. Doing so helps us better understand and love others, including ourselves. It also clearly focuses our energy on achieving our goals. Family traditions are limiting or false when they hinder one's ability to love, understand, and succeed. Transcending any limiting aspects of your family's heritage increases your capacity to achieve your potential. When you are unable to love yourself, you are unable to love others. Because low self-worth sits at the core of a variety of dysfunctional behavior (for example, drug abuse, alcoholism, physical and sexual abuse, and other addictions), it is crucial to expose any limiting family teachings that may destroy your sense of worthiness.

Most limiting traditions are not consciously spelled out. Since most of what we communicate is nonverbal, families pass along what we call "non- purposeful teachings." You'd never hear someone say out loud, "In order to get love in our family you need to get straight As in school and keep a spotless room." But a parent who focuses on these things to the extreme may send the nonverbal message that a child who fails in these endeavors is not worth loving.

People who love and honor their ancestors often struggle to look objectively at their family patterns. Loving children and grand-children often fear uncovering something negative about their relatives. They may assume that doing so will make their family appear bad, when in fact their family is good. Discovering limiting family patterns doesn't mean you've established an agenda to criticize your heritage. Rather, it is a process to improve upon it.

Pay close attention to your family's attitudes, to the nonverbal messages that are sent when a child behaves a certain way. Are you passing down biases and prejudices? Or are you passing down love and acceptance? How do your actions influence your children's behaviors? And how are your behaviors influenced by your own parents' actions? Spend some time writing down the answers to these questions. Discuss them with openminded siblings, a spouse, or a friend. Simply pinpointing what behaviors and attitudes come from your family's history may be an eye-opening experience and a catalyst for change.

To Strengthen Self-Worth

Oil Protocol: Blend 2 drops each bergamot, fennel, frankincense, geranium, and ylang ylang in a glass vial.

Application: Apply to the core of the body or the bottoms of the feet.

Affirmation: I love and accept myself.

Society's Powerful Influence

Max Lucado's book *If Only I Had a Green Nose* (2002) tells the story of a community of wooden dolls who rush to modify their appearances according to the latest trends: "Everyone wants to look like everyone else. Sometimes it's square hats. Sometimes it's tall shoes. Why, last year the big thing was yellow ears. Now it's green noses. Everyone wants a green nose" (p. 5). These wooden dolls, made by the great toymaker Eli, were not designed to look alike. But, as Eli explains, "They think they'll be happier if they look like everyone else. . . . I made them different on purpose. Freckles, long noses, bright eyes, dark eyes . . . these were my ideas. Now they all want to look the same" (p. 7).

Expectations exist all around us. And some of the most powerful expectations come from society and the communities in which we live. Families can choose to let these expectations enter their homes or they can actively select which expectations seep in and which are blocked. Consider for a moment all the varied beliefs that exist in different communities throughout the world. Some cultures believe it's good to be friendly, while others actively teach the importance of being reserved and restrained in social settings. Some communities believe it's best to coexist with your extended family throughout life, while others promote spreading out and living in single-family homes. Some communities may believe it's better to be black than white, or Muslim than Christian, or European than American, or skinny than full bodied.

The truth is, whether we're fat or thin, stylish or not, fair skinned or dark skinned, there must be a place each of us can go to feel our inherent worth—the glory that has been part of us since our birth. Our worth is inherent, and must be discovered. The home can and should be the place where parents and children can be who they really are. Complying with the opinions of society in the quest for healthy self-worth can be very damaging.

The hope of our future depends upon our youth. If you're a parent, grandparent, or teacher and sometimes feel as though you have no influence over the media and social norms outside your home, remember this quote by William Ross Wallace: "The hand that rocks the cradle is the hand that rules the world."

If you want to change your family, or even the world, here's a thought: Did you know that if two people marry and have three children, and those three children marry and have three children, and the pattern of marrying and bearing three children continues for twelve generations, the resulting number of descendants is a staggering 3,188,643 people! Because most of what we communicate is nonverbal, and most of who we are comes from our experience in our homes and families, the greatest changes we'll ever make are the changes we make inside ourselves while living with, and enjoying relationships within, our own families.

How can we influence an improved generation of youth? Here are some suggestions for parents, grandparents, teachers, and loving, influential friends.

Trust them! Children are born with inner knowing and are often more in tune with what's right and best than parents realize. Usually, youth will naturally gravitate toward greatness if we trust them and allow them to be authentic, remove our own judgments and fears, and let their intuitive nature thrive and guide them. To support yourself in building trust in you, apply bergamot or Roman chamomile oils. To help your child strengthen trust, apply lemon, marjoram, or lavender.

See them! Parents and teachers frequently project their personal issues onto youth. A parent's fears can play out in the life of a child if a parent doesn't take the time to look at his or her child as a separate and individual being. Don't think of your child as a mini-you! Look at your child as an individual who can become whatever he wants, despite your weaknesses and failings. To strengthen your vision of your own purpose, use frankincense however you'd like on a regular basis—diffuse it, wear it, inhale it! The more you use, the better your personal vision. To support your children in seeing their highest and best self, apply melissa or rosemary on the back of the neck and/or the bottoms of their feet.

Listen to them! Don't be so caught up in what you're doing that you don't really listen to your kids when they come to you. Put down the smartphone, turn off the TV, and really listen. Remember that listening is more than hearing what is being said. Pay attention to the nonverbal cues your child puts out there. Children who are heard are more apt to keep the communication lines open—a critical factor in establishing and maintaining a healthy relationship. Amazingly, nature can help in the communication process. Lavender essential oil frees the tongue and helps truth to flow. It's considered the essential oil of communication. Melaleuca (aka tea tree oil) enhances auditory communication, helping people hear things more effectively and clearly. Use both these essential oils regularly for you and your children.

Validate them! After you learn to listen, validate what you hear. Children who receive frequent validation of their thoughts feel more confident and empowered to succeed. Validation is the key to overcoming any relationship block. When we feel validated, we feel loved and supported. This process is essential to supporting healthy growth and self-esteem. Applying a grounding blend of oils (try blending blue tansy, frankincense, rosewood, and spruce with carrier oil) will help you and your children lift your heads in courage.

Encourage them! Today, most of the information communicated in our world is negative or critical. As a society, we seem to miss this essential point—encouragement does far more good than any form of criticism, judgment, or negative influence. If you find yourself in constant criticism of others, reach for a bottle of white fir and rub a few drops of the oil on your person. To encourage youth, massage cinnamon mixed with a bit of fractionated coconut oil on the bottoms of their feet or diffuse into the environment.

Support them! Many youth today feel unsupported—either adults in their world don't do enough to sustain them, or they do too much, and consequently hinder their potential. Real support comes when the right balance is maintained. Know what your child can handle while still being successful. Then, maintain that balance. To relieve anxiety, take the edge of stress off, and support your electromagnetic fields, try making the grounding oil blend mentioned earlier (blue tansy, frankincense, rosewood, and spruce with a carrier oil).

Protect them! Healthy boundaries are essential throughout life. Teach youth to stay away from destructive influences that will literally ruin them—and stop them if they head down a destructive path. Adults don't let two-year-olds play in a busy road for good reason! There are many dangerous influences that threaten the lives of youth, and keeping kids away from them is just as important as removing a baby from a busy road. Diffuse and apply wild orange and frankincense to help put on your armor and keep you protected and safe from the negativity of the world.

Guide them! Share your experiences and learning with youth and teach them correct principles that will foster long-term success. Even the kid who thinks he knows it all will usually listen to a parent who really wants to guide him and takes the time to share experiences and advice. A joyful blend of oils (try lavandin, lemon, melissa, sandalwood, tangerine, ylang ylang together) frees up inner wisdom to know the right things to say to your children.

Accept them! Remember in first grade when you colored a picture and thought it was a masterpiece? If you saw it now, would you think it looked like a Rembrandt? Probably not. Youth will often do their best, but still fall short of your expectations. They are still children, after all. They don't have the years of learning and expertise that parents do. We all learn by making mistakes, and healthy youth make a bunch of them. When you see a toddler throwing a fit, just smile and say, "He's perfect at being two." It really is okay when a teenager acts like a teenager and a wiggly boy acts rambunctious. Diffuse citrus oils regularly, as they help children and adults accept themselves.

Love them! Living all these tips in relationships sends a loud message that you love your family! Ultimately, that's all you can do to support anyone—and it's the best thing you can do. Love unconditionally without fail. Rose or eucalyptus, rosemary coupled with lemon, black pepper coupled with lime, or bergamot coupled with sandalwood all support our ability to love ourselves and others. Rub these blends on the back of the neck, the throat, or on the bottoms of the feet, then inhale by cupping your hands in front of your mouth.

CHAPTER FIVE

Intentions Rule

A touching scene in book two of Lucy Maud Montgomery's beloved *Anne of Green Gables* book series shows Anne embracing a sorrowful six-year-old Davy, whose attempt at playful mischief has gone horribly awry. Anne, a mischief maker at heart herself, knows a penalty to be necessary but understands Davy's innocent intentions:

> *"Punishments are so horrid and I like to imagine only pleasant things," said Anne, cuddling Davy. "There are so many unpleasant things in the world already that there is no use in imagining any more."* (1990, p. 90)

If one sentence can sum up the wonderful world created by Montgomery, it's that one. Anne Shirley—orphaned as a young girl and adopted by a stern old maid and her brother—overcomes adversity and childhood pains to grow up adored, smart, successful, and happy.

Part of her secret is how she combines her intention to be happy and her wonderful imagination, which has had readers in tears and stitches for well over a hundred years.

For Help with Transition and Change

Oil Protocol: Mix 3 drops each Roman chamomile, thyme, vetiver, and white fir with 1 drop of a commercial grounding blend (or make your own grounding blend with 2 or 3 drops each blue tansy, frankincense, lavender, rosewood, and spruce) in a glass roll-on bottle.

Application: Roll on top of the foot between the big toe and the index toe within the natural ridge. Next, roll on the back of the neck on the occipital triangle, and then declare your heartfelt affirmation out loud. If you sense personal resistance to change, add 2 drops melissa under the tongue.

Affirmation: I am capable of allowing change and I feel happy and peaceful about the changes in my life. (Repeat clearly 4 times.)

Montgomery, like her character Anne Shirley, grew up on Prince Edward Island. A relative's farm, named Green Gables, inspired the setting she imagined for her renowned books. Today, the town of Cavendish hosts most of the tourists wanting to jump into the imaginary world of Anne and become a little more like our redheaded heroine: optimistic and full of happiness.

The mind is a powerful tool, and the way we focus our attention and our intentions can make or break our lives. Whatever we focus on expands. The ideas that were once in Montgomery's mind alone developed into tangible elements as she expressed them in words and nourished them. Even though *Anne of Green Gables* is a fictional story, there is now an existing village in Cavendish that depicts the town of Avonlea, home to Anne, Marilla, Matthew, Diana, Gilbert, Rachel Lynde, and more. Her thoughts became reality, and consequently they inspired others.

Walt Disney spread a similar kind of happiness throughout the world with the development of myriad fictional characters that have become household names for most. But the imagination is not limited to fictional stories and characters! Many great inventors, writers, and leaders have changed the world by focusing on amazing ideas that have in turn enriched and blessed others.

We each have agency over our own thoughts and can choose both *how* and *where* to focus our energy. That focus typically defines our underlying intentions. Positive thoughts and good intentions tend to produce growth and healing, while negative thoughts and intentions tend to hurt and destroy. Take personal responsibility to use your power over thought wisely and effectively. The truth is, if the fruits of your thoughts and intentions make others healthier, happier, and wiser, then you are focusing your mind and efforts in a good, positive direction.

If you are filled with fear and doubt, it becomes an emotional challenge to shift gears from negative thinking to positive thinking and realign your intentions in a positive direction. But it is possible. Sometimes, just a simple reminder of the following important truths can turn around a sour disposition:

- First, you have the power to change your focus—you are worthy and capable of creating something good.
- Second, dreams do come true when you believe in them and yourself, and then take the time to create them.
- Third, dreaming is a good thing! It's healthy to use your imagination and focus your attention on your dreams, hopes, and happy living.

It's easy to be inspired by nature, and for Montgomery, Prince Edward Island was certainly a gorgeous conduit for a creative genius. Montgomery was said to find peace and inspiration during her walks through nature. Like Anne, she sometimes entered the forest in deep despair and came out invigorated and happy. Similarly, most of us could spend silent time somewhere in nature and reconnect our minds and hearts to the rhythm and beauty of our existence. Right now, as you're reading, consider how you're using your imagination. Are you focusing on thoughts of worth—ideas that heal, inspire, or serve? Are your underlying motives worthy of positive results? Do you find yourself feeling lovable, deserving, and worthy? If not, it may be difficult to create positive results until you make some changes within.

I Want to See More Stars

Becoming conscious is the process of bringing to full awareness the underlying emotions, thoughts, motives, and intentions that govern behavior. Harville Hendrix, Ph.D., psychologist and author of *Getting the Love You Want*, shares the following analogy, which can help us understand our consciousness:

> *In the daytime, we can't see the stars. We talk as if they "come out" at night, even though they are there all the time. We also underestimate the sheer number of stars. We look up at the sky, see a smattering of dim stars, and assume that's all there is. When we travel far away from city lights, we see a sky strewn with stars and are overwhelmed by the brilliance of the heavens. But it is only when we study astronomy that we learn the whole truth: the hundreds of thousands of stars that we see on a clear, moonless night in the country are only a fraction of the stars in the universe, and many of the points of light that we assume to be stars are in fact entire galaxies. So it is with the unconscious mind: The orderly, logical thoughts of our conscious mind are but a thin veil over the unconscious, which is active and functioning at all times. (1988, pp. 8–9)*

Most of us are trained to look at ourselves in a way that is similar to our observations of the universe during the daytime: We know we have a few issues (stars) that come out occasionally (at night), but we don't pay attention to them when we can't see them or understand them. Simply put, many of us aren't fully aware of our thoughts and our intentions. As we come realize that there is much more to us, just like there is much more to our universe than the view of stars seen in the daytime, we have a greater ability to heal.

What Did You Say?

There's wisdom in the adage that teaches "the most important thing in communication is hearing what isn't being said."

A general for the Union during the Civil War, Thomas Neill, said, "Of those who say nothing, few are silent."

In the same vein, poet Kahlil Gibran said, "The reality of the other person lies not in what he reveals to you, but in what he cannot reveal to you. Therefore, if you would understand him, listen not to what he says but rather what he does not say."

In our contact with others, we tend to focus primary attention on the information we consciously transmit and absorb. Many falsely assume that if we haven't said it, we haven't communicated it. While that may seem reasonable, it simply isn't true. Why? Because much of what we communicate is nonverbal. According to some research, up to 90 percent of our communication can be transmitted without words (Mehrabian, 1972). If we get stuck focusing on the words we hear (or say), we may miss the point—and unless we get the point, we may have trouble understanding, loving, and getting along with others.

Often we send (and receive) conflicting messages. For instance, we may say, "I love you" to our family members or loved ones. But if our actions communicate something different, those we love will not "feel" what's being said. Because what we "feel" is more powerful than what we hear, our actions can become the predominant form by which we communicate our love.

Often we're not honest when we communicate. We profess our love to others consciously, when inside our minds we're judgmental, angry, and unkind. We think we're hiding our negative intentions, hatred, or anger. In reality, we aren't hiding anything. All of what we communicate, even the data hidden in deep compartments inside our minds, gets transmitted.

If your associations with others lack healthy and functional communication, go back to your intentions. Most of the time, those who struggle to communicate effectively in their relationships have issues loving and accepting themselves. When we cannot be honest with ourselves about our fears, our past, our dreams, and our truth, we are not happy. The consequences ripple into our ability to communicate love in our relationships.

To Facilitate Clear, Nonverbal Communication

Oil Protocol: Blend 1 drop each basil and clary sage.

Application: Apply to temples.

Affirmation: I know I am loved; I see it in everyone around me. I communicate clearly and I surrender to the truth that everyone is loving and lovable.

The Law of Attraction

Once there was a man—let's call him John—struggling immensely with his marriage and his wallet. He was fired from his job, his home entered foreclosure, and his wife wanted a divorce. While his world seemed to be falling down around him, he wondered why his years of positive affirmations and visualization were mounting toward such seemingly negative drama. He asked, "Why am I creating exactly the opposite of what I want?"

That's a good and important question that many ask after learning and applying the Law of Attraction, a theory that basically describes how "like attracts like" and how positive thinking attracts positive results and vice versa.

There's a deeper reason John attracted the challenges he faced. John came from a broken home and grew up in poverty, often wondering where his next meal would come from. He married a woman with a similar background. Because of the challenges of his youth, deep down, John believed he didn't deserve to receive abundance or joy in his life. This engrained perception left John attracting situations where he would subconsciously validate his believe that he somehow wasn't privileged enough to receive the blessings he prayed for and attempted to manifest on a regular basis.

Generally, when we struggle to create abundance in our lives, whether it's a great flow of money or more love in our relationships, hidden feelings of being less than others or undeserving of blessings and goodness leave us unknowingly sabotaging our success, or simply not attracting it.

To Accept Wealth and Abundance in All Areas of Life

Oil Protocol: Blend 4 drops wild orange, 3 drops frankincense, 2 drops cinnamon bark, and 1 drop rose.

Application: Diffuse or apply on hands and breathe deeply. You can also rub on bottoms of feet.

Affirmation: I choose to live a healthy and happy life. Wealth flows easily and effortlessly to me. I celebrate my goodness and I am deserving of all that is good. I joyfully contribute to the goodness of this world. I fulfill my commitments and responsibilities confidently and with ease. Others appreciate and respect me. I am important!

In his book *The Power of Intention,* Wayne Dyer, Ed.D., gives this answer: "The law of attraction is this: You don't attract what you want. You attract what you are."

Dr. Dyer says, "Most people's mistake in trying to apply the law of attraction is they want things; they demand things. But God doesn't work that way—it's all about allowing" (in Griebel, 2008).

Sometimes, in order to attract the very things we want, we need to change something within ourselves so that we can become the kind of person (and energy) that will attract our greatest wish. Because deep, personal change can be brought about through personal trials and challenges, it's not uncommon for those who seek something new in their life to unknowingly manifest personal struggles as part of their learning process on the road to self- transformation. Often, we can misjudge our circumstances (or other's life challenges) as failures and further evidence of trouble, when, in fact, sometimes ill circumstances are a sign of personal transformation.

Dr. Dyer likes to share ancient teachings from Lao Tzu when he describes how to effectively work with the law of attraction. Dyer, following Tzu's lead, teaches that those who want to know the truth of the universe should adopt four basic virtues:

1. *Reverence for all life.* This manifests as unconditional love and respect for oneself and all other beings.

2. *Sincerity.* This virtue manifests as honesty, simplicity, and faithfulness.

3. *Gentleness.* This virtue manifests as kindness, consideration for others, and sensitivity to spiritual truths.

4. *Supportiveness.* This shows up as service to others without expectation or reward.

Many religions, cultures, and great teachers share similar philosophies. Interestingly, these same philosophies hold up in studies on human behavior and are values that define happy homes, successful marriages, and productive businesses. It seems that those who succeed in all areas of life, naturally share all, if not most, of these values.

To really get what we want most, we need to be searching inside our hearts and minds for personal shifts that bring us to forgiveness, acceptance, unconditional love, and service. Knowing this, it may be easier to see why, for some, it's a bit more challenging to apply the Law of Attraction.

Finding Success with Intention

As you seek to apply the Law of Attraction (or the Law of Intention) in your life, look at ways you can find success in creating a limitless future of joy and endless possibilities that are good.

First, realize that your energy field is complex and takes into account a broad variety of data, including the energy of family beliefs and traditions (which are often part of your genetic patterning), your quantum psychology (which consists of your mental and emotional makeup, including your belief systems, desires, fears, and self-definition), and your spiritual goals/divine purpose. All too often, conscious desires conflict with this complex and powerful energy source you hold within your body/mind. Resolution of the conflict comes through self-discovery and personal growth, which is a lifelong process.

After years of experimenting in the lab and with clients, we have discovered that Mother Nature—in the form of essential oils, particularly—can fuel the process of meditation and self-discovery necessary for personal success. Here are six steps, listed with complementary essential oils (apply one drop of each on the bottoms of the feet), to help you find success with the Law of Intention:

1. *Express your stored emotions.* (Cypress, eucalyptus, and wild orange free the tongue to express.)

2. *Uncover unhealthy desires, fears, and beliefs.* (Basil, geranium, and lavender encourage healthy exploration.)

3. *Discover your worthiness.* (Fennel, frankincense, and lemon clear and open the mind.)

4. *Find your real motive.* (Rose, melissa, and any citrus oil promote energy and vitality to move forward.)

5. *Harness destructive habits through consistent, uplifting, daily living.* (Lavender, marjoram, and oregano add balance and consistency to life.)

6. *Choose to love, forgive, and serve one another.* (Lime, rosemary, and ylang ylang promote peaceful and happy feelings.)

Think about this: If you were to hold up a clear bottle of purified water and add in a cup of dirt, what would the water look like? Murky, right? Would it make your water more clear and clean if you added a cup of fresh, distilled water to it? No. So it is with manifesting. When we add the good stuff (positive thoughts, affirmations, and consistent meditations) to a system that's already polluted with limiting emotions, fears, beliefs, and attitudes, we are diluting the situation. Resolution comes by cleaning out the system—which involves self-awareness, lots of self-expression, full transformation, and more.

Keep It Simple

Albert Einstein is presumed to have said, "Everything should be made as simple as possible, but not simpler." This is a great secret of happy living: realizing goals, projects, and purposes (including the missions of our lives) in an uncomplicated yet effective and prevailing fashion—eliminating the unnecessary while holding on to the essential details.

American writer Richard Bach is quoted as saying, "The simplest things are often the truest." Making it simple may come down to living a few basic, true principles. The suggested oils that accompany these principles may be used individually, diffused, or applied on bones behind the ears, while reflecting on your new good feelings.

Maintain focus. Keep your eye on the ball! Indecision breeds procrastination, and the two create huge distractions. You can hit only what you aim at. Outdoorsmen always "sight in," or adjust the aim of, a gun before hunting. Your goals should be no different. It requires regular focus to hit them. To gain focus, consider cassia, geranium, lavender, or lime—oils that are grounding and help one transition out of denial and move forward in a simple fashion.

Be honest—always! Nothing will make your life more complicated than lying—either to yourself or others. Facing circumstances squarely may seem challenging, but it's the simplest way to live a healthy and happy life. Remember, honesty is what you say to yourself, and not always what you say to others. If you lie to yourself long enough, you may come to believe it. Try frankincense or wild orange to promote honesty with yourself.

Prepare. Everything you need or want has a way of showing up as soon as you are ready for it. The sooner you're prepared, the faster you'll realize results. Some essential oils—such as basil and lemon—work to clear out the toxic fog in your system, fog that prevents you from keeping it simple. Try one of these or a cleansing blend made of cilantro, citronella, lemon, lime, melaleuca, and pine to help you talk less and accomplish more.

Have faith. Hopeful wishing is an excellent starter, but a not-so-good finisher. It is faith coupled with perseverance that leads you across the finish line. Faith comes after hope. It is believing without doubt! Experiment with myrrh or sandalwood to balance your head and heart and bring you home to truth, which leads to faith.

To Promote Faith Not Fear

Oil Protocol: Blend 4 drops sandalwood, 2 drops coriander, 1 drop ginger, and 1 drop wild orange with 2 tablespoons fractionated coconut oil in a glass roller bottle.

Application: Wear as a fragrance or inhale from the bottle as needed.

Affirmation: I am full of faith. Faith in myself. Faith in my future. Faith that I am on a journey meant only for me. I am positive and full of energy that radiates from me and positively affects others.

Keep it positive. Negative energy, feedback, and focus complicate everything! The three things you have full power over are your thoughts, words, and actions. Use them for good. Try bergamot, vetiver, and wild orange (for women), or white fir (for men) to stroke positive thoughts and diminish negative thinking.

Stay educated. Knowledge is a key that unlocks the door to dreams. Your individual success will depend upon increasing intelligence. Remember, all education is self-acquired—no one can really teach you without your permission to let their words in. You must choose it! Lemon, peppermint, and sandalwood support integrating knowledge.

Be courageous. Breaking out of old, complicated patterns takes guts. If your purpose is worthy and your pursuit is sincere, with bravery you can establish behavior patterns, thoughts, and choices that feed simple, happy, and successful lives. To support courage, create a blend of essential oils, mixing 4 drops helichrysum, 3 drops Roman chamomile, 3 drops sandalwood, and 2 drops lavender. Place blend on the bones behind the ears, along the throat, and on the lower back. This process helps the mind quiet fears, opens the heart to simple truth, and supports moving forward.

Go the extra mile. When you are spiritually compelled to reach out and serve (which we all are at one time or another), do it with high definition! It's a universal truth that leads to victory: What you put out comes back to you a hundred fold. Serve—and go the extra mile. You can use geranium, grapefruit, or white fir to support you in this process.

Drop the ego. You can't become the master of anything until you become the master of your own ego. While believing in yourself is important and healthy, inflating your sense of self by competing—or acting and believing you're better than others—will complicate your life in ways you cannot image. If your success is ego based, your failure is imminent. Love others instead and aspire to race only against yourself. Use 3 drops each of cypress, frankincense, and lavender on the forehead and neck. When applying, draw a "T" on your forehead, stroking the forehead across and then down along the nose. This helps clear the mind and calms the heart.

Be willing to work. Psychologist Virgil James used to repeat a popular saying, "With all thy get—get going!" Healthy self-esteem grows with good old-fashioned hard work, and anyone who's truly hit his mark will tell you that dreams aren't made without it. Frankincense is a wonderful oil to move you to honest and doable action.

We create complex lives and inherit difficult problems when we defy these straightforward truths that make for simple success.

As we work to improve our lives, it would serve us to evaluate our ability to live these truths. It may seem like an overwhelming list, and if that's the case, pick just one item and spend the week focusing on it. How do we eat an elephant? One bite at a time. So it is with living a balanced, healthy, and happy life—simplify the path to success by making one principle of success a part of your everyday life. Over time you will create what you want by adding in more principles, one "bite" at a time.

To Boost Courage

Oil Protocol: Blend 4 drops thyme, 3 drops fennel, 1 drop black pepper, 1 drop ginger, and 1 tablespoon fractionated coconut oil.

Application: Apply to bones behind the ears and the backs of the knees.

Affirmation: I am joyous and full of courage. I look to the future, live in the present, and let go of the past.

CHAPTER SIX

Courage to Change

A lbert Einstein said, "The significant problems we face cannot be solved at the same level of thinking we were at when we created them." What does this mean? In a nutshell, it means that problems are created by limited thinking and solved by elevated thinking. Elevated thinking requires change—in our minds, our hearts, and our perceptions. It also takes courage. A grand example of this is the great Italian physicist Galileo Galilei, who was once condemned—even rejected by society—for seeking to elevate thought on astronomy and physics. Today, Galileo is considered the father of modern science. And his elevated thinking has, indeed, answered many questions that remained unresolved as those around him resisted changes to their own limited thinking.

Like Galileo, we are each capable of initiating change. Sometimes, dramatic changes occur by simply adjusting our perceptions to include more possibilities. For example, on one occasion a man expressed his desire to work through barriers that had prevented him from purchasing a new home. The man lived in an expensive area and couldn't seem to qualify himself for a loan. After self-introspection, the man became aware of ways he had sabotaged his finances and thus his ability to purchase a house. Within three months of changing his perceptions, the man purchased a new home: He manifested his dream by changing himself.

To Foster Courage

Daytime Oil Protocol: Blend 4 drops Roman chamomile, 3 drops white fir, 2 drops bergamot, and 2 drops helichrysum in a glass vial.

Nighttime Oil Protocol: Blend 3 drops Roman chamomile, 2 drops clary sage, and 2 drops lavender.

Application: Rub 3 drops of blend on the back of the neck (base of head).

Affirmations: I am allowing my courage to lead me to what is best for me. I trust myself to handle what is in front of me. I am excited to manifest my own positive thoughts on what is next for me. I have the courage to change. I am embracing change with enthusiasm.

Change is a powerful tool—and it's really the only constant in our world. Whether we want to admit it, we're always changing and evolving. Charles Darwin is credited with saying that it's not the strongest that survive, nor the most intelligent, it's the ones who adapt to change the best.

When you can see new possibilities, you can create them. But to get to that point, you must be willing to move forward, despite obstacles. For many, the first obstacle to change is fear. Fear is a natural, human instinct. As such, it makes sense to turn to natural remedies for fear, specifically those found in nature and the essence of plant oils. Many essential oils—anise, caraway, coriander, fennel, ginger, peppermint, and tarragon, to name a few—have soothing properties that do everything from clearing the mind to tempering stomach acids and nerves. Blending these oils together makes a marvelous digestive oil that helps settle nerves and upset stomachs. Use the blend internally to support your body during times of change. Add one or two drops of each oil to an eight-ounce glass of warm water or tea and drink up.

In addition to fear, physical challenges—like panic attacks—can also become obstacles to change. Big changes can leave you feeling short of breath, anxious, overwhelmed, and stressed. Sometimes, these physical feelings can prevent you from pushing forward with change. When panic strikes, there are specific essential oils and breathing techniques that can be applied to reduce stress and help you move positively through changing circumstances.

We particularly like this application: Apply 2 drops lavender essential oil to the sternum in an upward motion toward the bottom of the throat, followed quickly with 2 drops eucalyptus essential oil. Next, place three to four drops wild orange essential oil on the inside of the forearms and rub together. This will do several specific things: The lavender and euca-lyptus will immediately relax the chest and support deep breathing. The wild orange on the forearms will soothe the heart and cause better cel-lular oxygenation. After applying these essential oils, take several slow, deliberate deep breaths. Together, this process provides clarity and re-laxation, leaving you free to choose a new way to react.

To Prevent Panic Attacks

Oil Protocol: Blend 4 drops geranium, 2 drops black pepper, 2 drops laven-der, 2 drops melissa, 1 drop frankincense, 1 drop wild orange, and 1 drop ylang ylang with 4 teaspoons fractionated coconut oil in a glass roller bot-tle.

Application: Apply to the sternum and back of the neck 3 to 4 times daily while focusing on the affirmation that follows.

Affirmations: I am fully competent and able to make good decisions for myself. I am safe. I am the only one thinking the thoughts in my head. I am capable of planning well and executing my plans successfully.

Mother Nature is very supportive of change and can be our best friend in times of transition. After all, it's Mother Nature that is the master and powerful creator of change! Consequently, walking out-doors in nature is often healing for those dealing with big life shifts. Most outdoor activities, even weeding a garden, can be relaxing and supportive. Physical exercise in nature, eating well (particularly lots of fresh fruits and vegetables), and getting sleep (a chance to balance yourself with the natural rhythms of the earth) all help individuals to transition well during change.

As you may expect, a positive attitude is helpful too. When your focus is negative, your chances for a positive outcome are reduced. Knowing this, it only makes sense to stay positive, despite potentially disastrous circumstances. Why not increase the odds of a happy ending by keeping a positive outlook? Wild orange and frankincense support a positive attitude. Place a drop of each in your palms and breathe the aroma in deeply. Rub remaining amounts on the throat and the back of neck. Repeat as often as needed.

Patience, trusting yourself, and staying true to your basic values and purpose are also important. When big changes throw them for a loop, many people find themselves on destructive paths because they've lost sight of who they are, where they came from, and where they are headed. There are essential oils that can help with clarity and purpose. Frankincense essential oil combined with Roman chamomile and cypress is helpful for mental clarity and emotional stability.

Finally, it takes courage to change. There are at least three types of courage:

- *Mental courage*: strength to venture, persevere, and withstand difficulty or fear.
- *Physical courage*: strength in the face of physical pain, hardship, death, or threat of death.
- *Moral courage*: strength to act rightly in the face of popular opposition, shame, scandal, or discouragement.

By applying courage to life's transitions, you will be equipped to move forward in a healthy and happy way.

Because every thought we have creates our future, dealing with our fears and eliminating doubts is an important part of transitioning well during times of change. The English poet William Blake once wrote, "If the Sun and Moon should doubt. They'd immediately go out."

When we begin to doubt—our dreams or ourselves—it can feel like the light within us has been put out. Doubt has the power to destroy hope, eliminate faith, halt growth, and blacken the future. And yet, on the flip side, a healthy amount of questioning can also bring wisdom. Albert Einstein said, "The important thing is not to stop questioning." Questioning can be good, as it leads us to examine ourselves and our dreams. The answers you receive when you question motives and processes can be productive and help you determine that you are on the right path. Questioning helps reassure you've selected dreams that support your highest good.

However, once you've resolved that your goals are solid, productive, and worthy of your labors, doubt can become a destructive voice. When this happens, respond kindly to yourself by listening, learning, and replacing your doubts and fears with positive, productive truth.

When you pay attention to the destructive, doubting voice, you come to understand more about yourself—and what you learn may be invaluable! Because you can't change what you don't know, coming to understand the reasons you doubt yourself is important. Next time you start to doubt and question, listen to what those doubts are saying. Then, to help clear your doubt, use ylang ylang, grapefruit, and white fir. Mix several drops of each oil together and apply to the sternum in an upward motion toward the top of the throat. Know that destructive doubt can set you up to sabotage your own success. Choose instead to uncover and conquer the very fears that are preventing your success.

Healing fears and false core beliefs by understanding what is true, enables us to replace lies (that we're bad and not good enough) with healthy beliefs (that we're worthy and deserving). Healthy beliefs breed healthy thoughts, and positive thoughts help us turn dreams into reality.

Remember, the body/mind is like a powerful, high-tech computer. Running old software—or running and rerunning old thought patterns and beliefs through the brain—leaves us limited to the capacity of the old program. If what we want to change—if what we want is something different than what we have (or something different from what our families taught us to have)—we must learn more about our programming and possibly replace it with newer, more productive and accurate information.

The Heart-Mind Connection

In a quiet place inside the mind and heart rests a still, small voice—an inner-knowing genius. It's not the part that adds, subtracts, and multiplies. It's not the logical mind that reasons and deducts. It's somewhat abstract and always accurate. It's intuition. And by listening to it, you can solve some of the most difficult problems that exist in your life. You can be guided to know simple things, like where you placed your car keys and which direction you should follow when you're lost.

Happiness, transformation, and inner peace come to us only when a solid connection is drawn between the heart and mind—when we look within. Inside of every human being exists the possibility for greatness. Tapping into your potential is crucial to success. Sadly, "Most of us have been enculturated during maturation to accept and believe certain things that may, and likely do, limit our real potential," writes Eldon Taylor, Ph.D., a fellow with the American Psychotherapy Association and the author of *Choices and Illusions* (2007, p. 13). Dr. Taylor's research indicates that each and every one of us has profound capacity. That potential is often denied due to the vast amounts of negative information we process each day.

According to Dr. Taylor, for every unit of positive information we process, ninety units or more of negative information are received. In other words, for each time we are praised, we receive ninety contradictory messages. Consequently, we find ourselves trapped in self-limiting beliefs about our abilities, intelligence, and worth. What we think and believe about ourselves determines our sense of well-being, sound health, and happiness—so understanding the influence of this critical input is essential to healing.

When we do not feel good about ourselves, we seek to find value and worth from others. Often, deep down we fear that we're worthless. Most of the time, we aren't necessarily conscious of these fears. Even so, they guide our behavior by pushing us to want and need the approval of others and leave us desperately fighting to comply with the rules of social conditioning. If we are caught in this cycle, we may be afraid to emotionally connect (or feel our real value) for fear we may discover we're worthless (an illusion). An indication of our participation in this cycle is easy to recognize: if we're judgmental and unjustly critical or harsh toward others or ourselves, or we find it difficult to connect in loving relationships, at some level, we're blocking our divine, internal connection to truth and wellness. Conversely, if we easily model charitable love (both toward ourselves and others) and we find it easy to connect in healthy relationships, learn, grow, give, and receive, chances are our minds and hearts, and our emotions, are connecting in positive ways.

Powerful personal change comes to us when we make that intuitive connection, bridging the body and mind and growing into a deeper sense of purpose. Practice makes perfect. The more we listen and respond to the inner voice, the better we become at hearing it. The better we hear it, the more apt we will be to transition well in life.

To Support Intuitive Connection

Oil Protocol: Blend 5 drops wild orange, 4 drops frankincense, 2 drops clary sage, 2 drops lavender, and 2 drops peppermint.

Application: Sweep around your body's core, along the sternum, and along the throat to the bottom of the chin.

Affirmations: I trust myself to listen consistently to the intuitive voice within me.

Science and Agency

As human beings, we have the power to choose our responses in every situation, and our responses are individual. In the foreword to *Healing Your Family History* (Hintze, 2006), Stephen R. Covey, MBA, Ph.D., shared the following.

While on a sabbatical many years ago in Hawaii, I was wandering in a reflective state through the stacks in a library. I pulled from the shelves a book containing three sentences that profoundly affected many aspects of my life and, particularly, my work. The sentences are these:

Between stimulus and response, there is a space.

In that space lies our freedom and power to choose our response.

In our response lies our growth and our freedom.

I reflected on those sentences again and again. I could hardly think of anything else for a period of time. I realized that between anything that has ever happened to us in the past—such as our genetic makeup—and our current circumstances is a space in which we can choose to respond. The outcome of that response can bring freedom and growth. Even though I intellectually understood this idea, the emotional force gave me both an exhilarating sense of freedom and a fearsome sense of responsibility.

In the gap between stimulus and response, we have the powerful opportunity to exercise agency. Agency is the ability to think, reason, and change. Nonetheless, our most natural response is to react according to instinct and prior conditioning, as though we were animals. But animals don't share our freedom of choice, intelligence, and capacity for transformation.

Unless we allow the soul—the human part of us—to guide us in the commitment to change, we may struggle to change our patterned behavioral responses.

Supporting our ability to release our natural, instinctive programming are essential oils such as sandalwood (its chemistry writes new information and patterns for our cells), lime (it allows us to change with positive expectations), grapefruit (it helps us to resist old patterns), and frankincense (it supports the balance between heart and mind).

To Facilitate Letting Go

Oil Protocol: Blend 3 drops each of frankincense and geranium with 2 drops each of myrrh and rose, 1 drop helichrysum, and 1 teaspoon fractionated coconut oil in a glass roller bottle.

Application: Dab on the forehead, neck, and temples. Repeat regularly.

Affirmations: I am accepting changes as they come. I am focusing on the great things that lie ahead of me. I am letting past hurts stay in the past and focusing on forgiving myself and others.

We Are Living Examples

It is through our examples that we impact others in both positive and negative ways. Clients often ask, "How do I get my spouse to change?" Or, "How can I help my children to change?" According to Albert Einstein, "Setting an example is not the main means of influencing another, it is the only means." Ultimately, it is through our examples that we impact those we love. There really is no other effective way to lead, teach, and train.

That makes us living examples—for good or bad. It's easy to forget about the lasting implications of our examples. Most of us don't think others are watching or believe that others notice our actions and responses or the things we might be privately stewing about. But remember, much of what we communicate is nonverbal. That means it really doesn't matter what we say, as much as it matters what we do, think, and believe. Every part of us is communicated in some form or fashion; and so, to truly influence others, we have only one course of action—to focus on ourselves and our own responses.

Ralph Waldo Emerson is credited with saying, "What you do rings so loudly in my ears that I cannot hear what you say."

As living examples, we have the opportunity to support growth and change in those we love. One way to do this is to seek to find the good within ourselves and model healthy self-worth. When we do this, we find we're less critical, more accepting, and kinder to family members. To further influence others, we can see the good in those we love. Often we put the light right out of our family members by continually casting our negative perceptions upon them. By focusing on the positive, we set the tone for our relationships. We can literally guide our interactions and craft them to be loving and kind by holding ourselves in a higher light, and then directing others to see us and them in the same positive way.

Supporting our ability to feel good about ourselves are essential oils like basil, bergamot, lemon, and ylang ylang. Apply them to the core while focusing on heartfelt positive intentions. When you want to positively influence others, apply these oils on your throat region and on the bones behind your ears.

We can influence those we love by modeling kindness and love. It's always a good idea to make a mental note of our own good qualities on a regular basis. Then, it becomes easier to focus on the positive characteristics of those we love. Pay attention to how your example influences positive behavior in your world.

CHAPTER SEVEN

Forgiveness Is Freedom

Forgiveness is a road to freedom—one that literally heals marriages, homes, hearts, and even crime in our communities. Consider the following:

- A twelve-month study on forgiveness and conflict resolution in marriage demonstrated that "Husbands' forgiveness predicted wives' current reports of better conflict resolution. . . . [And] over a 12-month period, wives' forgiveness predicted husbands' later reports of better conflict resolution controlling for initial levels of conflict resolution" (APA, 2006, p. 9)

- A forgiveness therapy model developed by researchers at the University of Madison-Wisconsin "has been shown to reduce anxiety and depression and to improve self-esteem in random controlled experimental trials" (APA, 2006, p. 11).

- A 2001 study examining physiological effects of rehearsing hurtful memories and nursed grudges found that those with "unforgiving thoughts prompted more aversive emotion, and significantly higher corrugator electromyogram (EMG), skin conductance, heart rate, and blood pressure changes from baseline" (van Oyen Witvliet, et al, 2001). Even into recovery periods, those with unforgiving thoughts demonstrated higher EMG, skin conductance, and heart rates.

- A 1995 study conducted by the University of Montgomery analyzed how an unforgiving heart factors into crime. The study showed that forgiveness plays a significant role in reducing the revengeful responses that prompt criminal acts.

To Facilitate Forgiveness of Self

Oil Protocol: Blend 3 drops of a grounding blend (try blue tansy, frankincense, rosewood, and spruce blended together) with 3 drops of a calming blend (try lavender, Roman chamomile, sandalwood, vanilla and ylang ylang blended together).

Application: Place in the palm of the hand and rub directly around the belly button, while stating affirmation and forming clockwise circles. Expect to feel different.

Affirmations: I forgive myself for believing misinformation about myself communicated by others. I forgive myself for denying my gifts and talents. I forgive myself for repeating destructive patterns and expecting a different outcome. I am free of criticizing, condemning, and judging myself. I release the past and live happily in the present.

If forgiveness can work miracles, healing hearts, minds, and bodies, why do so many of us resist it for so long? The answer is easy: pride. We are afraid that letting go means we are weak. And because forgiveness typically comes after being hurt, beat down, and damaged, the last thing we want to do is seem weaker.

In reality, forgiveness means strength. Charlotte van Oyen Witvliet, a professor of psychology at Hope College in Michigan, said: "Forgiving doesn't mean ignoring an injustice or letting someone treat you badly. Remember that it's not a wimp's response. It takes a strong, courageous effort to make that move. Letting go of your grudges takes a great deal of moral muscle" (2000).

To Facilitate Forgiveness of Others

Oil Protocol: Blend 3 drops each bergamot, geranium, helichrysum, melissa, and ylang ylang in a glass bottle.

Application: Place 3 drops of blend in hand and rub counterclockwise around the belly button while stating affirmations out loud.

Affirmations: I forgive others for their inability to recognize that I have needs. I forgive others for communicating false information about me. I am free of criticizing, condemning, and judging others. I communicate only loving messages to and about myself.

Mahatma Gandhi taught, "The weak can never forgive. Forgiveness is the attribute of the strong."

In addition to strength, there is honesty in the process of forgiving. A real recognition of the pain of the offense, coupled with a strong desire to love and let go, allows forgiveness to occur. The truth is, if we really want to love, we must get to the point where we're strong enough to forgive. While we cannot change others, we can change the way we feel about our past, and even ourselves. In the process of forgiving, we enhance the present, change the course of our future, and halt the negative trends of history that tend to seep into the future.

While forgiving others is a necessary step down the path of freedom, so is forgiving ourselves. All too often we carry the burdens of our past and refuse to let go of our mistakes. We get caught in a never-ending cycle of negativity when we hold on to self-condemnation and use it to punish ourselves. When we're penitent and apologetic of our past and restitution has been made, forgiving ourselves is the final step in healing.

Practice forgiveness! It is your key to freedom. If you find that you're offended, sad, or depressed about pains from the past, seek relief through the miracle of forgiveness.

Once again, we suggest turning to nature in your quest to forgive. Examining nature itself can provide a wealth of information about forgiveness. Just think about the harshness of winter and how spring follows mercifully with a forgiving heart and the promise of new life. As you examine nature, take the opportunity to use its elements as well. Among the essential oils that calm and encourage balance and forgiveness are frankincense, lavender, marjoram, rosewood, sandalwood, spruce, vanilla, and ylang ylang. Rub these oils on the center of the body while making the statements, "I forgive myself for not being perfect. I am free of past mistakes. I am free to be me."

To Relieve Hurt and Bitter Feelings

Oil Protocol: Blend 2 drops each helichrysum, lavender, and rose with 1 teaspoon fractionated coconut oil.

Application: Apply over liver.

Affirmations: I am letting the sweet take over the bitter. I am choosing to be better instead of bitter. I don't let misinformation about myself trouble me. I know who I am and I am happy with who I am.

Sheri Dew, CEO of Deseret Book Company, writes, "Though we must each walk through life on our own, we don't have to do it alone" (2003). Do you realize how powerfully significant our associations with one another are? We either influence and support others for good or we provide help that is not so good.

Sometimes in the field of self-help, we push the concept of *interdependence*—or the process of being emotionally sound through self-reliance. According to Webster's dictionary, interdependence implies that all participants are emotionally, economically, and/or morally "independent." It's a great concept; however, it doesn't stand alone.

This is because we live in a world where one affects the whole—it's a fact! One bad apple has the power to wipe out the bushel. One angry, irresponsible, and abusive adult (or leader) can leave a lasting imprint on the lives of those he abuses. Likewise, one loving, forgiving, and charitable family member or friend has the power to heal the lives of those he loves. In truth, it's not reasonable (or honest) to expect ourselves to become so self-reliant that we are no longer dependent on relationships or no longer affected by the actions of others.

Interdependence flies out of balance when self-reliance is used to push people away, create walls in relationships, or block love in our lives. We must learn to stand together as a part of the whole— not as an island. When we can't receive what we need from others, two things typically happen to us. First, we suffer because we are left to do without the love that we need to survive. And second, we suffer because we are no longer giving love to others; and forgiveness and charitable giving are necessary parts of our emotional survival too.

We all want and need to be loved and we all need at least a few key friends and family members to walk with us along the road of life. When we start feeling like this isn't the case, it becomes important to assess our situation. Like Miss Clavel in the popular *Madeline* stories, hold your forefinger to the wind and say, "Something is not right!"

What's not right? Here are a few possibilities:

- You may have been so badly hurt by someone that you don't trust others enough to receive their love. When this happens, many people tend to use self-reliance to protect themselves from their fear of rejection.

- You may be so afraid you're not as good as others that you push people away because you fear you're not lovable anyway.
- You may be afraid to fail in your own ability to love and forgive, so you don't try.
- You may be sad that others don't see your heart—and thus fear wrongful judgment or criticism—so you don't try.
- You may have grown up in an abusive home environment and have no idea how to love and forgive others.

Notice how many times "fear" is mentioned in the preceding list. It's true that fear is typically the biggest block keeping us from forgiving and enjoying loving relationships.

Consider how well you stand together with others. Are you enjoying the blessing of companionship as you walk the road of life? If not, ask yourself why. How can forgiveness help? If your fears block you from giving and receiving love, search inside for ways to eliminate these blocks. If you're not attracting a healthy support system, begin today to make changes inside so that you may stand together with others you love as you walk through life. Take time daily to apply the essential oil protocols that assist with forgiving to support such changes.

Essential Values for Successful Families

Successful marriages and families are established and maintained when families incorporate values such as forgiveness, respect, love, and compassion. When families engage in behaviors that are highly destructive (like abuse, addiction, codependency, critical sarcasm, gossip, ridicule, judgment, and overuse of guilt), family members find themselves either holding on to grudges because of their pain, or having the opportunity to learn and exercise forgiveness. Despite the painful circumstances of our youth, forgiveness can offer us a new start—a chance to be free of the anguish and pain we may recall from years past.

To Break Free of Patterns of Codependency

Oil Protocol: In a glass vial, blend 3 drops of a commercial massage blend (or make you own with basil, cypress, grapefruit, lavender, marjoram, and peppermint), 3 drops of a respiratory blend (made with eucalyptus, laurel leaf, lemon, peppermint, and tea tree oil), and 3 drops each geranium and oregano.

Application: I allow myself to grow beyond my family patterns. I am free to be me. I deserve. I take responsibility for my life.

Abuse and codependency are big things that require a lot of work to forgive and heal. Codependency occurs in families when children believe the parents' needs are more important than their own. Abusive parents generally create codependent children. Parents who struggle to be responsible for their lives and themselves often leave behind a generation of youth who don't know who they are and feel out of control. By accident, codependent personalities become obsessed with control, not realizing they have a choice over the course of their lives, because they never felt important enough to have a choice! Once a codependent pattern is recognized, those who grew up with these sorts of patterns may find themselves angry and unhappy with their parents.

What's true is that despite the difficult circumstances of our youth, we have the freedom to choose to move forward through forgiveness. Generally, every parent is doing the best they can in their lives. While parents and grandparents may unknowingly (and sometimes knowingly) pass on destructive patterns, their worth as souls is still inherit and deserves forgiveness.

That kind of forgiveness is big and takes some work. But even the little things need forgiving if we really want to break the cycle and start a new tomorrow. To live healthy and happy lives, we must learn to forgive everyone who may have wronged us. We must forgive those who've taught us ineffective ways to think, behave, and believe. We must forgive the people we blame for causing us sorrow or making us doubt. Why? Because when we can't forgive, we naturally hold on. Holding on causes more pain; it enables wounds to fester and promotes separation from those we love. But forgiveness is a powerful tool. It is, in fact, a blessing. There is nothing more rejuvenating than a heart full of forgiveness, ready to overcome the mistakes of the past, be they small or profoundly serious.

As you implement forgiveness in your families, the natural re-sults will be a home full of more respect, kindness, and compassion. And these are certainly values worth passing on to those you love. After years of research, a study about kindness and unkindness in families showed that the single most important ingredient in a happy home is kindness. The study found it is not kind tasks that do the trick, it is kind people—and there is a difference (Burr et al., 2012).

People who are charitable by nature and concerned with the long-term welfare of others in thought, word, and deed, will con-tribute to the long-term happiness of the family. To some it may seem old-fashioned to speak of these values—forgiveness, respect, love, and compassion—but these are the qualities which have built great families. Even today, they point the way by which one may find happiness. These are qualities that act as anchors in our lives, despite the trials, the tragedies, and the cruelties that can leave us suffering. The truth is: We cannot be happy without them.

The German poet Friedrich von Schiller wrote:

Wouldst thou know thyself, observe the actions of others. Wouldst thou other men know, look thou within thine own heart. (1871)

A client once said, "I feel I am able to love my husband, my chil-dren, my ancestors, and my friends and neighbors—why? Because

I've gained self-respect, I've forgiven—so much that I can say that I've truly learned to love myself."

To Enhance Creativity and Follow-Through

Oil Protocol: Blend 3 drops helichrysum, 2 drops basil, 2 drops clary sage, 1 drop rose, and 1 drop wild orange with 3 tablespoons fractionated coconut oil in a glass bottle.

Application: Add 2 to 3 drops of blend to the palms of hand and rub together, then inhale.

Affirmations: I receive inspiration and divine guidance daily. I complete my projects and goals with creativity and inspiration. I am directed, divinely guided, and loved.

The Solution

Every problem has a solution. These are wise words taught by many experts, including best-selling author Louise Hay. In 2006, Louise turned eighty years old. At her birthday celebration in her hometown of Carlsbad, California, just before blowing out the candles on her cake, Louise gave some short, sweet advice. She said, "Forgive yourself, forgive everybody else, cut out the crap, and love who you are!"

Louise has spent years offering solutions to hurting hearts, minds, and bodies. She's written countless articles and books and has sold more than 50 million copies of her work. Where does her wealth of wisdom originate? Like all of us, Louise has access to higher knowledge and truth. Louise knows that solutions come from within. Whatever problems we're facing, answers can be found by listening and learning from divine intuition. Through meditation and prayer, we can access just the solutions we need.

Louise's simple message of forgiveness and love is perfect! When we seek to love ourselves and others enough to truly forgive, we find that our minds become hopeful and open to new and enlightening information. When we "cut out the crap" we let go of negative influences that limit our growth and happiness. And when we embrace and love who we are, we are happy and much better equipped to contribute positively to the lives of others.

It's a Wonderful Life

During the Christmas season, the classic movie *It's a Wonderful Life* airs regularly on television, reminding viewers of the far-reaching effects of one person's life. In the movie, a depressed George Bailey (played by actor Jimmy Stewart) believes his life is worthless. He wishes he had "never been born," and to his surprise, an angel gives him his wish come true in a dream, where he sees what the world would be like if he'd never existed and interacted with anyone. Marvelously, George realizes the influential impact of his seemingly ordinary life (one ridden with mistakes). Like George Bailey, it's easy for each of us to forget the impact our lives have on the whole, despite our weaknesses and errors.

We are valuable, important people—every one of us! Marianne Williamson, spiritual activist and best-selling author of *A Return to Love*, reminds us of our glory.

Our deepest fear is not that we are inadequate. Our deepest fear is that we are powerful beyond measure. It is our light, not our darkness that most frightens us. We ask ourselves, Who am I to be brilliant, gorgeous, talented, fabulous? Actually, who are you not to be? You are a child of God. Your playing small doesn't serve the world. There's nothing enlightened about shrinking so that other people won't feel insecure around you. We are all meant to shine, as children do. We were born to make manifest the glory of God that is within us. It's not just in some of us; it's in everyone. And as we let our own light shine, we unconsciously give other people permission to do the same. As we are liberated from our own fear, our presence automatically liberates others. (1996, pp. 190–91)

It has been said that when we lift ourselves, we lift a great many others at the same time. As we are busily engaged shining our light, our world changes. It is through forgiveness that we free ourselves to the point where we recognize all that is good in ourselves and others.

We will all have days when we feel like George Bailey at his lowest. When you do, it helps to let go of your fears and remember the love you've given away throughout the years and how that love has affected others. In the process, you will find that your life has value and beauty.

Imagine you are George Bailey—shown by angels the value and influence of your life. Forgive yourself and let yourself see the good you've contributed. As you do so, the influence of your life will continue to expand, and you will find that "It's a wonderful life!"

CHAPTER EIGHT

Love It!

What is love?

In *The Story of My Life,* Helen Keller tells the touching story of how she came to understand love's meaning:

I remember the morning that I first asked the meaning of the word, love. *This was before I knew many words. I had found a few early violets in the garden and brought them to my teacher. She tried to kiss me; but at that time I did not like to have any one kiss me except my mother. Miss Sullivan put her arm gently round me and spelled into my hand, "I love Helen."*

"What is love?" I asked.

She drew me closer to her and said, "It is here," pointing to my heart, whose beats I was conscious of for the first time. Her words puzzled me very much because I did not then understand anything unless I touched it.

I smelt the violets in her hand and asked, half in words, half in signs, a question which meant, "Is love the sweetness of flowers?"

"No," said my teacher.

Again I thought. The warm sun was shining on us.

"Is this not love?" I asked, pointing in the direction from which the heat came, "Is this not love?"

It seemed to me that there could be nothing more beautiful than the sun, whose warmth makes all things grow. But Miss Sullivan shook her head, and I was greatly puzzled and disappointed. I thought it strange that my teacher could not show me love.

A day or two afterwards I was stringing beads of different sizes in symmetrical groups—two large beads, three small ones, and so on. I had made many mistakes, and Miss Sullivan had pointed them out again and again with gentle patience. Finally I noticed a very obvious error in the sequence and for an instant I concentrated my attention on the lesson and tried to think how I should have arranged the beads. Miss Sullivan touched my forehead and spelled with decided emphasis, "Think."

In a flash I knew that the word was the name of the process that was going on in my head. This was my first conscious perception of an abstract idea.

For a long time I was still—I was not thinking of the beads in my lap, but trying to find a meaning for love in the light of this new idea. The sun had been under a cloud all day, and there had been brief showers; but suddenly the sun broke forth in all its southern splendor.

Again I asked my teacher, "Is this not love?"

"Love is something like the clouds that were in the sky before the sun came out," she replied. Then in simpler words than these, which at that time I could not have understood, she explained:

"You cannot touch the clouds, you know; but you feel the rain and know how glad the flowers and the thirsty earth are to have it after a hot day. You cannot touch love either; but you feel the sweetness that it pours into everything. Without love you would not be happy or want to play."

The beautiful truth burst upon my mind—I felt that there were invisible lines stretched between my spirit and the spirits of others. (2004, pp. 25–26)

To Promote Positive Feelings

Oil Protocol: Blend 3 drops of a commercial joyful blend (or make your own with lavandin, lemon myrtle, melissa, sandalwood, tangerine, and ylang ylang), 3 drops frankincense, 2 drops bergamot, 2 drops myrrh, and 2 drops rose or geranium in a glass roller bottle.

Application: Dab on the forehead, around the ear, on the back of the neck, and along the throat; at bedtime, massage 2 to 3 drops on the top of each foot.

Affirmations: I receive inspiration and divine guidance daily. I complete my projects and goals with creativity and inspiration. I am directed, divinely guided, and loved.

If love is the invisible line connecting us together, are we really loving one another when walls exist that block loving connections? We all have the opportunity to overcome our fears of being loved and giving love. Doing so helps us experience what Helen Keller felt when she described her vision of love—a deep, spirit-to-spirit connection. Love is a divine attribute. Without it, we are not happy or fulfilled.

Love also requires responsibility. When he won the Nobel Peace Prize, Tenzin Gyatso, the Fourteenth Dalai Lama, said:

Responsibility does not only lie with the leaders of our countries or with those who have been appointed or elected to do a particular job. It lies with each one of us individually. Peace, for example, starts with each one of us. When we have inner peace, we can be at peace with those around us. . . . When we feel love and kindness towards others, it not only makes others feel loved and cared for, but it helps us also to develop inner happiness and peace. (1989)

Serve with Love

It's one of the basic laws of nature and a biblical and moral imperative: Give and you shall receive. But did you know that giving service to others is a basic human need—as important to our development as obtaining food and shelter? Today, psychologists emphasize this fact, reminding us that offering community service is a major factor in determining not only the happiness of individuals but also the success of families and nations.

A 1992 study of the effects of altruistic behavior on adults found that self-esteem and a sense of well-being increased (by as much as 24 percent) for those who served. In fact, it was simple acts of kindness that produced the reward—simple acts like holding the door open for others, thanking the mail carrier or doorman, and helping the elderly carry groceries. It takes only a small shift in attitude to produce positive results in our lives (Hafen et al., 1992).

Deepak Chopra, M.D., promotes seven laws of spiritual success, of which number two is the Law of Giving:

This law could also be called the Law of Giving and Receiving, because the universe operates through dynamic exchange. . . . The flow of life is nothing other than the harmonious interaction of all the elements and forces that structure the field of existence. . . . Because your body and your mind and the universe are in constant and dynamic change, stopping the circulation of energy is like stopping the flow of blood. Whenever blood stops flowing, it begins to clot, to stagnate. That is why you must give and receive in order to keep wealth and affluence—or anything you want—circulating in your life. . . . In order to keep that energy coming to us, we have to keep the energy circulating. . . . The more you give, the more you will receive. (1994)

Perhaps Dr. Chopra's evaluation explains why in two major studies on volunteerism, "healthy-helper syndrome" was identified as a side effect of giving without expecting anything in return. This type of sacrifice and giving with a deep concern for another resulted in reduced arthritis pain, fewer lupus symptoms, and in a reduction in the number of asthma attacks, migraines, colds, and the incidence of flu (Hafen et al., 1992).

It's true that serving one another in an honest way supports healing—both physically and emotionally!

Be Thankful

There are times in life when each of us has the wind knocked out of us and, through hardship, the light within our souls is challenged. Often it's through the brightness of another that the weakened spirit is rekindled. The deep appreciation that fills our hearts when we are the beneficiary of love and service is gratitude. Universally, we've all been blessed in countless ways.

To Promote Gratitude and Joy

Oil Protocol: Blend 4 drops bergamot, 3 drops wild orange, 2 drops rose, and 2 drops white fir with 1 tablespoon fractionated coconut oil.

Application: Apply to bones behind ears. Put in hands and rub together, then inhale deeply.

Affirmations: I am grateful. I fill my mind with heartwarming thoughts of gratitude. I allow joy to fill my entire being. I am taking the steps I need to take to be grateful and happy in my mind, mood, and thoughts.

Gratitude helps us grow. It brings us joy and happiness. And as we express it, we bless the lives of all those around us. A French proverb says, "Gratitude is the memory of the heart." It has also been said that gratitude is not only the greatest of virtues, but it is the parent of all the others. Author and speaker Anthony Robbins said, "When you are grateful, fear disappears and abundance appears."

Is it possible that becoming grateful is the answer to overcoming fears and living happy lives? A good many experts agree—the answer is yes! Gratitude is high-frequency energy. It attracts all that is good. When we're thankful, somehow, miraculously, life works for us.

Can we be grateful for everything and everyone? Absolutely. Even the villains of our lives offer us gifts of knowledge, peace, and reconciliation. A movie without a villain is boring, and a life without challenges and enemies is dull as well. By developing an attitude of gratitude and giving thanks for everything that happens, we are better able to move forward in life, realizing that every step forward is a step that helps us obtain something bigger and better.

If you're feeling like you need help being thankful, pick up a notebook or a blank sheet of paper. Place it in a convenient and noticeable place. Every time you have a chance, jot down what you're able to recognize that's good in your life at the moment. Maybe you're thankful for your soft pillow, a warm and sunny day, a home-cooked meal, or an opportunity to read a good book. Focus your thought energy on the good things in life—all you have to be thankful for. Look for opportunities to be a light of love and strength to those who may be suffering. As you do so, you'll find yourself having one of your very best weeks.

The Law of Least Effort: Acceptance

Dr. Chopra's fourth law in *The Seven Laws of Spiritual Success* is to accept people, situations, and events as they occur. How does this formula make for an easy and happy life?

First, by accepting people, situations, and events as they occur, we surrender our need to control others. Think about it. What happens when we don't accept people, situations, and events as they occur? We generally wind up trying to control them! Many have learned, from trial and error, this universal truth: It's impossible to control others and almost impossible to control most situations.

And "control" is the opposite of "freedom." When we want to be free, we mustn't control.

Pastor Reinhold Niebuhr made famous this useful prayer.

God grant me the serenity to accept the things I cannot change, the courage to change the things I can, and the wisdom to know the difference.

Second, when we take responsibility for our lives, we are no longer held hostage by the past; the present views, opinions, and actions of others; or our fears about the future. Many mistake the real meaning of "taking responsibility" and associate it with carrying a burden, guilt, and blame. When we take responsibility, we take charge of our emotions and forgive. We like to think of forgiving as literally giving back (or "fore" giving) to others the responsibility they may have inappropriately placed on us through wrongdoing. By forgiving with love, we allow ourselves freedom to move forward. And we give those who've hurt us the opportunity to heal. This helps everyone!

Last, when we relinquish the need to defend our point of view, we can rest easy. In so doing, we gain confidence, strengthen self-worth, and solidify our godly purpose. When we can stand firm in the truth of our divine selves, we are ready to serve our world in a profound way. It is by fulfilling our purpose through service that we gain the greatest joy in life.

To Release the Ego and Accept Ourselves and Others

Oil Protocol: Blend 3 drop cypress, 3 drops frankincense, and 2 drops lavender.

Application: Apply to forehead and neck.

Affirmations: I release my fears and I am safe. I allow others and myself to be wrong. I fully accept myself and others. I understand that I am perfect exactly the way that I am.

The Magical Healing Power of Love

Love may not seem like a treatment for health and emotional conditions, but the truth is that it's a powerful, abundant solution that is not only nontoxic to our bodies, but costs nothing and can be self-administered. So, why don't we refer to it more often as a legitimate health solution? Maybe because love isn't something we bottle or sell. It involves the wisdom of our hearts, and receiving it may mean we need to change ourselves, our lives, or our relationships.

Have you ever reached out to a loved one to serve and support them in a time of need and your efforts have been rejected or misrepresented? When hearts are emotionally blocked to love, healing with love is difficult to say the least.

Love shows up for us in numerous forms: embodied expressions like compassion, charity, respect, nurturance, empathy, reverence, concern, understanding, affection, gratitude, support. In fact, any kind of caring can feel like love.

Taking love in as a treatment can also feel like a connection to ourselves and the world around us. According to James Lynch, M.D., a specialist in psychosomatic medicine at the University of Maryland's School of Medicine, the more connected we are to life, the healthier we are. Dr. Lynch teaches that "Love your neighbor as yourself " is not just a moral mandate, but also a psychological *and* physiological mandate. He confirms research that thoughts and emotions become chemicals, and our positive thoughts and feelings (like love) release powerful endorphins in our bodies that act as natural painkillers and enhance mood as well as immunity (see Hafen et al., 1992).

Another interesting study that inadvertently demonstrated the healing power of love was conducted at Ohio State University by husband-and-wife team Ronald Glaser and Jan Kiecolt-Glaser. The study was intended to look at cholesterol levels in rabbits. Strangely, the results demonstrated that only half of the rabbits who were fed a high-cholesterol diet ended up with high cholesterol. The mystery of the unexpected results was revealed when the team discovered that a lab assistant had cuddled the bunnies that ended up having low cholesterol during the study because they were in the lower cages where she could reach them. She could only throw the food to the bunnies in the top cages, so she never touched them. The half that didn't develop high cholesterol was literally protected by the loving touch of the lab assistant!

Similar studies have produced results that demonstrate the power of caring for humans. These results have been documented in studies of premature babies, nursing home residents, burn patients, orphans, alcoholics, and people with tuberculosis, arthritis, and heart disease (see Ornstein, 1990).

To receive one of these love treatments, find a listening ear—someone who loves you and genuinely cares to hear you—and share your woes. Studies have shown that several immune functions are elevated in people when they express their feelings and confide in others who love them. If a human ear is unavailable, pets work well too (see Ornstein, 1990).

Even just observing loving actions around you may also be beneficial. The "observer effect" was coined after a Harvard University study tested volunteers' salivary immunoglobulin before and after viewing three films, including one on Mother Teresa and her work. After seeing the video on Mother Teresa, the viewers' markers improved by an average of 50 percent (see Ornstein, 1990).

Really, I could go on and on discussing the powerful truths about love and how it can be the magical treatment for humanity. The bottom line to all of healing may be just this—our ability to truly love ourselves and others. This may also mean loving the stories and the circumstances of our lives by coming to accept all that is good in the world around us.

As you seek permanent and lasting healing, we call upon all readers of this book to come closer to this powerful healer—love. As you do so, you will truly live a healthy, happy life.

To Experience Serenity

Oil Protocol: Blend 2 drops clary sage, 2 drops melissa, 2 drops wild orange, 1 drop lavender, 1 drop Roman chamomile, and 3 tablespoons fractionated coconut oil in a glass vial.

Application: Wear as a fragrance or inhale directly from the bottle as needed.

Affirmations: I am at peace. I am calm. I create serenity all around me.

Appendix

The standard guidelines for emotional wellness include consumption of a nutritious diet (with supplementation whenever needed), elimination of unhealthy foods and other substances from your diet and environment, adequate water intake, proper sleep habits, a resourceful outlook on life, and choosing to engage in respectful, supportive relationships. In addition, essential oils can have a positive emotional impact on you by elevating your mood, promoting relaxation, and contributing other health benefits.

This appendix contains an index of individual essential oils as well as of common oil blends you can purchase from various essential oil producers. Although these blends go by varying names, depending on the manufacturer, they typically contain similar oil mixtures. You can also make oil blends at home in proportions of your own preference.

Note: The descriptions here are provided for informational purposes only, as suggestions for the kinds of results individuals may experience. Your own results may vary.

Individual Essential Oils

Accompanying each entry that follows is general information about the oil, emotional states it may benefit, and suggested affirmations. The oils are listed alphabetically by their common names. *Note: Oils may be used aromatically, topically, and/or internally (when it is specified that it is safe to do so on the product labels on their packaging). Some require dilution with a carrier oil, such as almond oil, coconut oil, grapeseed oil, or jojoba oil, when they are applied directly on the skin.*

Arborvitae *(Thuja plicata)*. Arborvitae is a member of the tree family. It is grounding and stabilizing to the nervous system. Because it has antiviral, antibacterial, and antifungal properties, it protects and sustains those who use it. Arborvitae is a hearty plant that produces a high yield of essential oil. It may be used to support those who feel broken or ill due to relationships that have been abusive or where there are patterns of codependency. It can be helpful to those facing divorce. If you need additional resources to sustain your strength, better personal boundaries, and a stronger connection to life, arborvitae may provide that added support. It may leave you feeling capable, sturdy, grounded, powerful, and independent.

Emotions: Uncertainty, instability, fear, sadness, loneliness, agitation.

Affirmations: I am whole and healthy. I am confident and capable. I accept and love myself as I am. I am able to respond to my needs and the circumstances of my life in healthy and appropriate ways. I am centered and grounded. I am connected to life everywhere.

Basil *(Ocimum basilicum).* Basil is a member of the mint family. As an herb, it has strong medicinal properties, making it an excellent choice for the treatment of flu and infections. It can also be used to treat mental exhaustion and poor memory. Basil helps renew the mind and restore energy to the body. Its positive properties may help reprogramming the type of emotional patterns that underlie different addictions. Basil can restore hope to the soul.

Emotions: Anger, anxiety, stress, fear.

Affirmations: I am enough. I am peaceful. I release all fears and transform them to faith. I am safe and everything works out for me.

Bergamot *(Citrus bergamia).* A member of the citrus family, bergamot is an excellent choice for uplifting our moods. For those with low self-esteem, bergamot may help restore confidence, hope, and self-assurance. Bergamot supports us to let go of negative thinking and release tension. It also encourages us to connect to who we really are so we may share our authentic selves with others. Applied to the throat, solar plexus, and the bottoms of the feet, Bergamot can assist with a good night's sleep. When diffused, it helps create a peaceful environment. Combine bergamot with lime and sandalwood to promote a sense of worthiness and belonging.

Emotions: Self-doubt, discouragement, self-hatred, disappointment, discouragement, stress.

Affirmations: I love and accept myself. I love who I am. I am worthy and important, confident and capable. I am comfortable being me.

Birch *(Bentula lenta).* Birch is a member of the tree family. Distilled from bark, its properties are soothing for the soul as well as for pain and inflammation in the body. Birch is helpful for those who feel they are unsupported by the people around them. When we feel alone, birch can comfort us and provide us with strength. It offers sustenance by helping us feel rooted enough to face the storms of life. It also gives us sufficient buoyancy that we may stand alone. Physically, birch provides support to our structural systems—our muscles and bones.

Emotions: Fear, worry, pain, anger, instability, disconnection.

Affirmations: I am supported. I am grounded and stable. I am connected to my life's purpose. I release the past and make room for stable growth. I allow myself to be and feel comforted.

Black pepper *(Piper nigrum).* A spice with potent antiviral properties when taken internally, on an emotional level black pepper is helpful in eliminating the "virus" of negative thinking. It pulls up suppressed emotions so that they can be dealt with honestly, promoting recovery from addiction and encouraging new ways of thought. Black pepper helps us let go of the old and increases our capacity for the new. It may help those who bottle up emotions to release destructive feelings.

Emotions: Fear, anxiety, overwhelm, self-criticism, doubt.

Affirmations: I am free to choose. It is safe to feel. I am able to peacefully and fearlessly face the truth of my past and my present, and my feelings about it. I accept that I am healing one day at a time.

Cardamom *(Elettaria cardamomum).* Made from seeds of a plant in the ginger family, cardamom has a refreshing and invigorating aroma. A versatile spice used in cooking around the world, it stimulates digestion and helps clear channels in the kidneys, making it a tonic for overall health. When we are physically well, our spirits are uplifted and our minds become clearer. Because cardamom stimulates blood flow, it has a warming effect. This effect helps clear congestion from the lungs and may also help overcome conditions such as impotence.

Emotions: Confusion, depression, grief, resistance, frustration.

Affirmations: I am focused and intentional in everything I do. My mind is alert and I am inspired to do great things. My actions are aligned with my best interests. I am able to envision a bright future.

Cassia *(Cinnamomum cassia).* Cassia is an oil of courage for those who are shy and hold themselves back. It helps rid us of fear and replace it with self-confidence by helping us recognize our talents and potential. Cassia is also medicinal in nature and can assist in helping those who feel overrun by life to regain inner strength. Cassia is high in cinnamaldehyde, and as such, has been shown to be useful for killing different strands of bacteria, particularly those associated with Lyme disease.

Emotions: Shyness, anxiety, self-doubt, timidity, overwhelm.

Affirmations: I courageously face my destiny. I enthusiastically share my gifts and talents with the world. I am safe to let others see and know the real me. My strength is building day by day.

Cedarwood *(Juniperus virginiana).* Cedarwood helps those who struggle to form social connections. It opens the heart so we may feel the love and support of others. It helps us to feel like we belong and rid our souls of impressions of loneliness and isolation. Cedarwood belongs to the conifer tree family, and as such, it's soothing to the central nervous system. Consequently, cedarwood can be used topically on the bottoms of feet along with lavender and/or Roman chamomile to support a good night's sleep. It is also purifying and sedative.

Emotions: Depression, anxiety, irritability, confusion, loneliness.

Affirmations: I am calm and secure. I am safe to connect. My heart opens to receive love. I am deeply supported. Life is on my side.

Cilantro *(Coriandrum sativum).* Cilantro is a type of parsley. It comes from the same plant as coriander, but is extracted in a different way— by steam distillation from the leaves. High in antioxidants that protect our cells from oxidative stress, it also helps us cleanse ourselves of the negative emotions that weigh down the body. It's a natural detoxifier, physically and emotionally. It can help us interrupt patterns of ridged, destructive behavior and lighten our emotional load, allowing us to return to our true selves. Cilantro may be supportive for migraine headaches and riding the body of heavy metal toxicity.

Emotions: Rigidity, resistance, self-hatred, irritability, anger, stress.

Affirmations: I am in flow. I am effortlessly releasing thoughts and feelings that do not serve me. My mind and heart are untouched by negativity around me. Positive energy uplifts me unceasingly.

Chamomile, Roman. *(See Roman chamomile)*

Cinnamon *(Cinnamomum zeylanicum).* Distilled from bark, cinnamon essential oil is a spice oil that is helpful in regulating blood sugar. It has antibacterial and immune-boosting properties. It promotes well-being by supporting healthy digestion. Emotionally, it restores joy and supports sexual health. It encourages us to be honest and vulnerable in our relationships, allowing intimacy to flourish, while also supporting us in sustaining healthy boundaries. It also has been known to rekindle desire that has been lost due to trauma or abuse.

Emotions: Depression, mental exhaustion, post-trauma, low libido.

Affirmations: My mind is sharp and my body healthy. I am able to set and sustain healthy personal boundaries with the people in my life. I am able to trust myself. I allow myself to experience intimacy.

Clary sage *(Salvia sclaria).* Clary sage is a member of the mint family. It promotes clarity of mind and helps us to open our psyches to new ideas and perspectives. It supports creativity by increasing our ability to focus and visualize. It can also help us better develop our spiritual gifts. Physically, it interacts with the body's hormonal system, and can therefore bring hormonal balance and stimulate interest in intimacy. Women entering menopause may find it useful to combine clary sage with geranium (topically) to support mood and hormonal balance.

Emotions: Mood swings, disconnection, depression, low libido, stress.

Affirmations: I trust myself completely. I remain calm, cool, and collected at all times. I am a powerful creator. I am focused and persistent. My mind and my heart are aligned with my intentions.

Clove *(Eugenia caryophyllata).* Clove is a powerful antioxidant that has many medicinal uses, including the treatment of toothache, digestive upsets, parasites, and arthritis. Emotionally, clove supports us in establishing healthy boundaries in relationships. It gives individuals with a tendency to feel victimized and helpless to control what's going on around them a sense of personal power and control. It supports us in being able to do what is necessary to protect ourselves.

Emotions: Fear, helplessness, overwhelm, anxiety, self-doubt.

Affirmations: I am confident and capable. I am in charge of my destiny. I believe in myself and my abilities. Everything works out well for me.

Coriander *(Coriandrum sativum).* Coriander oil comes from the same plant as cilantro, but is distilled from the seeds. Coriander is an excellent support for those of us who are people-pleasers or who have lost sight of who we are and can't find joy in the lives we've created. It is also especially useful for emotional eaters. Emotionally, it teaches us that we can be happy as we are and do not need to repress our emotions. Often, we grow up believing we must please others to be loved, and thus, happy. When there is no joy in life, at times, we may turn to sugar and sweets to make us feel better. Coriander supports us in being loyal to ourselves by encouraging us to do the things that are in alignment with the true self. Physically, coriander is helpful for blood sugar imbalances. A therapeutic-grade drop of coriander may be taken internally to support the body when there's been too much sugar intake. It's also useful to rub coriander directly over the pancreas.

Emotions: Sadness, flatness, instability, anxiety, suppression, anger.

Affirmations: I allow myself to feel my feelings. I love and accept myself. I affirm my right to stand my ground when people disagree with me. My needs are always taken care of effortlessly.

Cypress *(Cupressus sempervirens)*. Cypress oil supports the free flow of energy. Individuals who feel emotionally stuck may find cypress a great resource. It encourages us to be more flexible and let go of control. It's also tremendously helpful for bringing up and then releasing deeply stored pain. As a member of the tree family, it provides emotional grounding. Physically, cypress is supportive to the circulatory system—improving the flow of blood and lymph. It strengthens the structural systems of the body: bones, muscles, and soft tissues.

Emotions: Loss, fear, resistance, uneasiness, trauma, depression.

Affirmations: I am flexible and free. I am grounded and centered. The energy of the universe flows through me and promotes the good of all. Obstacles in my path and around me are dissolving effortlessly.

Dill *(Anethum graveolens)*. An herb in the parsley family, dill promotes purification of the body, digestion, and healthy nervous system functioning. When we're in a heightened emotional state or being challenged, it can help us stay calm. In situations where we feel we are being unfairly treated or we are having a hard time accepting reality, dill oil can help us to "digest" or process our emotions successfully.

Emotions: stress, anxiety, depression, agitation, overexcitement.

Affirmations: I accept what is without feeling diminished in any way by it. I remain peaceful and relaxed always. I feel happy to be alive.

Douglas fir *(Pseudotsuga menziesii)*. A highly fragrant tree oil used medicinally by Native Americans and long associated with the celebration of Christmas, Douglas fir promotes mental clarity and creativity, and elevates our moods. It naturally revitalizes the spirits and soothes the soul. Douglas fir oil promotes healthy respiration and can also reduce muscular pain and stiffness—thereby making us feel good. When we use it, we experience a sense of general well-being. Those who tend to become scattered in their thinking or are easily distractible, due to ADHD or chaotic circumstances, find it restores their focus.

Emotions: depression, futility, loss, stress, mental fatigue.

Affirmations: My mind is alert and I am focused on my goals. I easily accomplish anything I set my mind on doing. My spirit is uplifted and I am filled with the energy for living. I love expressing my creativity.

Eucalyptus *(Eucalyptus radiata).* Eucalyptus has been used for centuries to support the respiratory system. In promoting easy breathing, eucalyptus supports healing and wellness. In particular, eucalyptus seems to tap into the emotions of those who have a pattern of illness and helps them move forward to living in wellness. It encourages us all to face our issues head on and let go of negative emotions. Eucalyptus is grounding and soothing to the soul and silently suggests a renewal of life and good health to an ailing body and spirit.

Emotions: anger, oversensitivity, grief, resistance, stress, frustration.

Affirmations. As I breathe, I sense all the obstructions in my life dissolving effortlessly. My soul is soothed as I remember to breathe. I am connected to the life force that animates everything in the universe.

Fennel *(Foeniculum vulgare).* Historically, fennel has been used to promote digestive wellness. It's also known to support hormonal balance. And just as fennel supports digestion, it helps us digest the process of life. It strengthens our souls to imagine that the desires of the heart can be obtained. Fennel supports us when we feel overwhelmed by reminding us of our potential, helping us reconnect with our inner selves, and inspiring remembrance of a bigger perspective.

Emotions: Stress, depression, overwhelm, frustration, fear.

Affirmations: I boldly step forward into my future. Everything I desire is mine. I deserve happiness and fulfillment. My potential is unlimited.

Fir, Douglas. *(See Douglas fir)*

Frankincense *(Boswellia frereana, B. carteri, B. sacra).* Frankincense is often referred to as the "father" of all essential oils because it has so many applications. This oil helps us to connect to our inner spirits. It helps rid us of spiritual darkness and mental deception by helping us see the light within and remember our talents and potential. It improves our attitudes and intuition. Also, frankincense reminds us that we are loved and not forgotten. Frankincense is helpful for anyone who is struggling with issues with a father, either temporal or spiritual.

Emotions: Fear, shame, disappointment, insecurity, self-doubt.

Affirmations. I trust myself and I remain calm at all times. I am safe. I am supported and unconditionally loved. My needs are being met.

Geranium *(Pelargonium graveolens).* Geranium soothes a broken heart and powerfully releases past baggage. It helps individuals who have lost hope in people and the world around them. Geranium reminds the soul that the world is mostly good and most people have good intentions. It also brings up the pain of the past so one can work through old emotions and begin to see all that's good. Geranium may be combined with clary sage to bring hormonal balance (and thus mood balance) to women during menopause. Combine with lime oil if you are working to release deeply rooted emotional wounds.

Emotions: Loss, disappointment, fear, depression, mistrust.

Affirmations: I am kind and patient with myself and others. The world is a safe place. I am patient with my healing process. Every experience gives me an opportunity to love myself and others more.

Ginger *(Zingibar officinale).* Ginger is the ultimate encourager. It helps us to live in the present and seize the day. It empowers us to achieve the potential we were destined to fulfill. Just as ginger oil promotes physical digestion, it encourages healthy digestion of uncomfortable challenges and supports resolution of gut-related anxiety.

Emotions: anxiety, stress, fear, obstinacy, doubt, complacency.

Affirmations: I am fired about my plans and ready to meet my challenges head on. I am present and alert. I love to express myself creatively. I am a powerful creator with an important destiny to fulfill. I digest the process of life. I am nurtured and supported.

Grapefruit *(Citrus x paradisi).* Grapefruit is a member of the citrus family, and as such, a natural mood uplifter. Historically, grapefruit oil has been used topically (diluted) to reduce fat from problem areas of the body because it cleanses toxins from fatty cells. Consequently, it is a great essential oil for individuals who are unhappy because they can't seem ever to be satisfied with the way they look. Grapefruit helps us love our bodies more by inspiring us to pay attention to what our bodies really need. It also may help control appetite. Because it can improve hormonal balance, it helps to eliminate "toxic" thoughts relating to self-worth. When combined with cassia and inhaled, grapefruit can increase our confidence in ourselves and our appearance.

Emotions: Self-hatred, dissatisfaction, negativity, depression, anxiety.

Affirmations: I love and accept myself as I am. I love my body. I am grateful to my body for providing my soul with a home on earth. I love moving my body and eating healthy foods that fuel my activities.

Hawaiian sandalwood *(Santalum paniculatum).* Hawaiian sandalwood is very calming and stabilizing. It harmonizes our emotions and gives us mental clarity and the intuition. Many people find that Hawaiian sandalwood enhances meditation.

Emotions: stress, anxiety, low libido, depression, lack of focus.

Affirmations: I am beautiful inside and out. It is comfortable for me to openly reveal my authentic self and express my truth. With every breath and every step, I increase my peace. All is well.

Helichrysum *(Helichrysum italicum).* Helichrysum is the ultimate essential oil for healing deep emotional pain, which it helps by addressing the emotions that are behind the pain. Helichrysum helps restore the love for living that individuals who have been weighed down by agony feel, because it encourages the restoration of belief. It is useful for those struggling with addiction when they experience self-rejection and self-hatred. It may be useful to rub helichrysum over the liver, as the liver is the organ that is traditionally associated with painful emotions like anger, fear, and hate.

Emotions: Anger, fear, hatred, depression, self-recrimination.

Affirmations: I release and I let go. I let Spirit/God run my life. I deeply forgive and fully accept myself for everything I was, I am, and I will be.

Jasmine *(Jasminum officinale).* Jasmine is a fragrant essential oil with a sweet scent that has long been associated with romance because the jasmine flower blooms only at night. Jasmine oil is pleasing and emotionally elevating, and may stimulate the release of serotonin and other hormones, resulting in a surge of energy and a sense of overall wellbeing. Jasmine opens the heart and paves the way for improved intimacy for couples who have grown distant, and it makes it easier for those who are drawn together out of attraction to trust one another. Jasmine oil is calming and may help promote undisturbed sleep. It is also good for the skin and for relieving self-consciousness.

Emotions: anxiety, disconnection, self-consciousness, mistrust, stress.

Affirmations: I am safe to love freely. I trust myself. I am open to new experiences. Sleep is my friend.

Juniper berry *(Juniperus communis).* Juniper berry is an excellent resource for the bladder and kidneys. It's often used to treat kidney and urinary tract infections. Emotionally, juniper berry helps those who are ridden by fear, anger, and a lack of security in life. Juniper berry suggests ways to the mind and body to work through the underlying issues that creating intense fear and anger. It helps one feel protected and have the courage to face life with the knowledge that it's possible to create peace, balance, and a sense of security.

Emotions: fear, anger, distrust, stress, grief, holding back.

Affirmations. I release that which no longer serves me. I am willing to forgive myself and others for being human. I accept that I am doing the best I can. I feel peaceful and protected. All is well.

Lavender *(Lavandula augustifolia).* Lavender is the oil of communication. It enhances cellular communication and also encourages honest communication. It helps individuals express their true selves. Lavender is a powerful anti-inflammatory. It is calming and soothing to the central nervous system and can dramatically help reduce symptoms of anxiety. It is sometimes considered the mother of all essential oils, offering some of the broadest medicinal uses, from treating burns and bug bites, to reducing joint pain and helping eliminate headaches.

Emotions: stress, agitation, anger, fear, anxiety, distrust.

Affirmations. I freely express my authentic truth. Opportunities are everywhere for me when I am ready. I am relaxed and at ease in every situation. I am at peace with my body. I accept and love myself as I am.

Lemon *(Citrus limon).* Lemon is a natural mood uplifter. Its clean, fresh scent lightens the environment and encourages cleanliness and emotional housekeeping. Lemon supports individuals who have learning disabilities or find it hard to focus. It assists us in finding clarity and choosing to live in the present moment, focusing on one thing at a time. It also restores confidence in those who have negative self-thoughts associated with learning. Lemon is also highly antibacterial and can be used as a natural hand sanitizer while uplifting mood immediately when inhaled.

Emotions: Self-doubt, anxiety, confusion, frustration, overwhelm.

Affirmations: I am capable of greatness. I am able and willing to learn. I love myself unconditionally. It is a joy to contribute my gifts and talents to the world. My future is bright. I am perfectly supported and nurtured to grow into my full potential.

Lemon balm. *(See Melissa)*

Lemongrass *(Cymbopogon flexuosus).* Lemongrass is a fantastic emotional house cleaner (assuming the body is the house of our emotions). It supports individuals who feel stagnant in life to clear the clutter and move forward. It helps energy to flow freely so we can live with confidence. Lemongrass can bridge the gap between desires of the heart and mind. Physically, it is helpful for bringing balance to the thyroid system. It's highly antimicrobial, anti-infectious, and helpful at increasing circulation, so it's often taken internally to promote wellness.

Emotions: fear, negativity, self-criticism, doubt, lack of drive.

Affirmations: When my intentions are clear, the universe cooperates with me and I can accomplish anything. I am always successful. Success is in my blood. Life is beautiful. Life is fulfilling. I love life.

Lime *(Citrus aurantifolia).* Lime, a member of the citrus family, lifts mood, supports the respiratory system, and helps individuals feel joy by helping rid negative emotions like depression and discouragement.

It instills love and happiness back into the heart. It's wonderful for releasing grief and pain. Combined with geranium, lime can wipe away the barnacles and clear the path, making way for beneficial change.

Emotions: anxiety, anger, depression, discouraged, mental fatigue.

Affirmations: I feel energized and uplifted by my life. Joy is my name and gratitude is the nature of my game. I am easily releasing negativity.

Marjoram *(Origanum majorana).* Marjoram relieves joint and tissue pain, particularly when combined with lemongrass. Alone, marjoram helps individuals who cannot create meaningful relationships, because of deep emotional wounds or trauma, to move forward and connect. Marjoram can assist in helping us learn to trust others and ourselves. It is a member of the mint family, and as such, it has antibacterial and antiviral properties making it medicinal in nature.

Emotions: anger, depression, self-doubt, anxiety, loneliness.

Affirmations. I am a good person. I am strong, courageous, and brave. I am not alone today. The trauma/abuse/betrayal was not my fault. I trust myself. My life has a beautiful meaning and a higher purpose.

Melaleuca *(Melaleuca alternifolia).* Melaleuca oil is also known by the common name tea tree oil. Melaleuca supports healthy boundaries. It's used medicinally to support daily wellness, reduce unwanted and destructive bacteria, and keep the body fresh and well. I have been chronically ill, Melaleuca rebuilds confidenc(good health. It supports us in creating strong boundarie rid ourselves of negative thoughts of others and ourselves. Melaleuca can help us desire to stick up for what we believe in and desire.

Emotions: anger, shame, fear, confusion, resignation.

Affirmations: I can see others' choices as learning experiences without judging. I allow others to experience their own lessons. I am a go-getter and will stop at nothing to achieve my goals. My body is my ally in living the wonderful life of my dreams.

Melissa *(Melissa officianalis).* Melissa is also known as lemon balm. Melissa is a powerful support to the human brain. It is also highly antiviral, and thus supports freeing the body of unwanted programming that affect healthy thinking. Melissa is sometimes referred to as the oil of truth. It helps individuals see who they really are and why they are here. It can support spiritual connection. It encourages one to press on through the hard times and love their life. It is a strong supporter of relieving depressive symptoms and recovering from traumas that have impacted the brain.

Emotions: disconnection, depression, trauma, anger, negativity.

Affirmations: Obstacles are now falling away easily. I have a right to my feelings. Today, I welcome health and happiness. I abandon old habits and choose new, positive ones. I am the authority on my own experience. I deserve love, success, and fulfillment in great measure.

Myrrh *(Commiphora myrrha).* Myrrh essential oil is made from the distilled resin and gum of a tree. It is an extraordinary preservative that was used by ancient Egyptians for embalming, and as such, is excellent for the skin. Myrrh oil balances the thyroid system, which regulates our metabolic processes; it also helps heal subconscious conflicts and encourages nurturing self-expression. It also supports healthy gums and mouth care. Just as myrrh can be used at birth to help heal the cutting of an umbilical cord of a newborn, it can help heal relationships, specifically a hardened relationship between a mother and her child. Myrrh helps the child within each of us feel safe and loved, filling any void in our mother/child relationship. Myrrh supports meditation.

Emotions: anger, shame, disconnection, depression.

Affirmations: I am in perfect communion with the wholeness of creation. I am completely true to myself, alive and empowered, fully and freely creative. I am sheltered by the mercy of spirit/God/the universe. I am divinely led and guided in all I think, do, and say.

Orange, Wild. *(See Wild orange)*

Oregano *(Origanum vulgare).* Oregano is a very powerful essential oil that can relieve pain and infection. It can get through to individuals who are stubborn and hold tightly to an unhealthy belief systems. It's strong medicinal properties work similarly to prescription antibiotics. Metaphorically, oregano works similarly on our emotional system, fighting convincingly for the body's sound emotional health by eliminating unwanted thoughts and patterns. Oregano makes a strong statement to let go of toxic attachments, bad relationships, and sabotaging habits, thus making it easier to move forward in life.

Emotions: obsession, resistance, negativity, competition, jealousy.

Affirmations: The more I focus my mind upon the good, the more good comes to me. I trust I am being led to where I need to be. My life is important. I can change the world just by being here, right now. I surrender my ego and no longer let fear and envy rule my life.

Patchouli *(Pogostemon cablin).* Patchouli is a grounding essential oil that helps stabilize the central nervous system. It fosters communication between the heart and body so that they can work better together. It also supports us in letting go of negative thoughts about life and reminds us to find beauty in the world around us. Patchouli can cross the blood-brain barrier to chemically support the brain and nervous system. Patchouli can aid in addiction recovery, as it works to shift our mindset and reestablish a healthy connection to life.

Emotions: anxiety, regret, self-doubt, worry, depression, insecurity.

Affirmations: I am surrounded by people who love and support me, and I love and support myself. I respect myself and know that my opinion and voice matter. I communicate my feelings and needs in healthy, respectful ways. My needs are met easily and effortlessly.

Peppermint *(Mentha piperita).* Peppermint stimulates the brain and increases circulation. To rapidly increase mood and brain function, combine peppermint with wild orange and inhale. As you do so, you'll find you've increased neuronal activity in your brain (you'll also open your sinuses and breathe more easily), and suddenly you'll feel a wave of happy emotions encompass you. Emotionally, peppermint helps individuals who are struggling with depression to see the joy in life. Peppermint helps to lift sadness and pressure and can put a cap on an overflow of unhealthy emotions. However, we should not use peppermint as a permanent escape. It should be used to help see the joy of life and encourage us to work through the issues holding us back. Peppermint is also good for headaches, memory, and focusing.

Emotions: Sluggishness, depression, stress, lack of focus, resistance.

Affirmations: I am open and receptive to all the abundance life offers me. I can handle massive success with grace. The positive advantage is always mine. My attitude grows happier and healthier every single day. I am focused and in flow. Happiness is my birthright.

Petitgrain *(Citrus aurantium)*. Made from the leaves of bitter orange, petitgrain essential oil is an extraordinarily potent mood elevator. It may help stimulate the mind, promote the recall of positive memories, reduce mental fatigue, and ease depression. The scent is vibrant and refreshing. When we use petitgrain it is like pressing the reset button on a computer screen and opening a new "window" for life to surprise us. Antioxidant, anti-inflammatory, antibacterial, and anti-infectious, as our immunity is boosted by petitgrain and we heal physically, our moods may stabilize and we may experience more joy at being alive.

Emotions: depression, irritability, lack of focus, confusion, fatigue.

Affirmations: My personality is radiant with confidence, certainty, and optimism. I am always in the right place at the right time. Today is rich with opportunities and I open my heart to receive them. I am joyful.

Roman chamomile *(Anthemis nobilis)*. Roman chamomile helps us feel calm and restores our sense of purpose in life. It is very calming to our minds and bodies, and help heal broken hearts. Roman chamomile also helps individuals who have lost their sense of who they are to regain their purpose in life. It gives us confidence and the motivation to succeed. Roman chamomile also promotes healthy digestion. For this reason, we know that it can help us digest the emotions we feel.

Emotions: grief, depression, purposelessness, fear, agitation, shock.

Affirmations: In my sadness, I love myself. All things are unfolding as they are supposed to. I let go of my sorrow, but hold on to my love for my loved one. I am discovering new strengths within myself.

Rose *(Rosa damascena).* Rose encourages spiritual healing by helping us feel divine love. When an individual can connect to divine love, emotional wounds tend to resolve. Rose helps us to connect to love by encouraging connection, prayer, and meditation. When we connect in this way, we often feel more compassion and charity. Rose restores clarity and reestablishes the power of a loving spirit to heal through love. Rose can be useful at both birth and death encounters, bringing great peace and comfort to these substantial transitions in life.

Emotions: disconnection, depression, fear, envy, grief, shame.

Affirmations: I live skillfully and effectively, and I am steadily awakening to self-realization. I constantly experience and express complete well-being in all aspects of my life. I am invincibly protected against any imperfect suggestion. I am the living embodiment of a divine spirit.

Rosemary *(Rosmarinus officianalis).* Rosemary encourages us to gain greater knowledge by searching for deeper answers. It helps to expand the mind beyond first assumptions. It also helps us feel comfort and confidence in times of change. Rosemary is helpful for adrenal fatigue and mental exhaustion. It helps the respiratory system, thus aids in lifting the burdens weighing heavily on us. It promotes detoxification.

Emotions: stress, anxiety, fear, depression, overwhelm, fatigue, grief.

Affirmations: The healing energy of the universe surrounds me and I am restored to perfect health. I am living my life according to my highest vision, which is inspired by love and joy. I am the architect of my life; I build its foundation and choose its contents. I am a radiant being.

Sandalwood *(Santalum album).* Sandalwood assists us in opening our souls to honest and healthy connection. In doing so, it offers clarity and spiritual strengthening. Sandalwood helps to calm the heart and prepares us to talk to God/our higher power. It also allows us to see life in a bigger perspective. It can help us better align our lives with divine purpose. Research on sandalwood suggests that it has powerful properties that aid in restoring healthy cellular function.

Emotions: confusion, regret, purposelessness, depression, stress.

Affirmations: My nature is divine. I am a spiritual being. Everything that is happening now is happening for my ultimate good. I love myself and I accept myself as I am. I am naturally feminine, graceful and beautiful. I am a woman of love. My touch heals all wounds.

Sandalwood, Hawaiian. *(See Hawaiian sandalwood).*

Spearmint *(Mentha spicata).* A member of the mint family, the menthol fragrance and taste of spearmint is refreshingly buoyant and rejuvenating. It may bring relief from depression and stagnation of energy.

Emotions: stress, anxiety, agitation, overexcitement, isolation.

Affirmations: The whole process of living makes me happy. I am grateful to God for this wonderful life. I am thankful to everybody who has touched my life and made it worth living. I am kind, I am loving, I am happy.

Spikenard *(Nardostachys jatamansi).* Spikenard essential oil has been highly prized for thousands of years in the Middle East and Far East for its far-ranging uses. Complex in composition, it is valued for its ability to foster regeneration of the skin. Emotionally, it assists us when we're in transition between different roles and identities, and undergoing rapid growth as people. Spikenard promotes higher consciousness and opens the third eye so that our powers of intuition may intensify.

Emotions: disorientation, anxiety, fear, resistance, lack of clarity.

Affirmations: Today I am blessed with absolute clarity. I am on purpose and achieving results. Wisdom guides my vision. I am an expert at keeping my thoughts in order. I feel confident and capable when surfing the waves of change.

Tangerine *(Citrus reticulata).* Tangerine essential oil is perfect for those who feel burdened by responsibilities that aren't theirs. From the citrus family, tangerine frees us to let go and be happy, to find the joy in life and escape debilitating pressures for a period. It also helps to replenish our creative juices. Tangerine is a natural mood uplifter.

Emotions: overwhelmed, fatigued, depressed, burdened.

Affirmations: My heart leaps with joy the moment my eyes open in the morning. I maintain a continuous attitude of gratitude. Joy is mine right here right now. I choose to be joyful, loving, and inspired.

Tea tree. *(See Melaleuca)*

Thyme *(Thymus vulgaris).* Thyme helps release emotions that may be buried deep down, including anger that's been stored for a long time. Bringing unhealthy emotions to the surface helps us process through them and ultimately get rid of them. By ridding our hearts, minds, and bodies of strongly rooted negative emotions, such as hate and resentment, we can create better health, confidence, and emotional fortitude. A member of the spice family, thyme is naturally antimicrobial. It is also a powerful antioxidant and analgesic.

Emotions: grief, depression, guilt, hatred, resentment, resistance.

Affirmations: Today is a clean slate. I am gentle with myself and others. I am smart and I can find a solution. My intentions are pure.

Vetiver *(Vetiveria zizanioides).* Vetiver is tremendously supportive for the multitasking mind that tends to gravitate toward symptoms of ADHD, such as distraction. It helps balance the mind and promotes clarity for those who feel torn between people and priorities, or struggle making simple decisions. Vetiver smells like the earth, and grounds individuals, helping them connect to their true selves. It encourages confidence to know what to do when, and why. It may be used to help restore a healthy sleep cycle, to support focus and attention during the day, and to release painful past trauma in the way of mental focus.

Emotions: mental fatigue, resentment, distraction, frustration, anger, trauma, stress, shock, depression, anxiety.

Affirmations: I share my opinions freely and easily shrug it off when someone disagrees. I commit to being honest about who I am and what I love. Making wise decisions is easy for me. My life improves every day and in every way because of my wise decisions.

White fir *(Abies alba).* White fir is a natural painkiller. It belongs to the tree family and so it is naturally grounding. Specifically, while fir helps to heal generational patterns and wounds. Emotions are passed down through family members, some that are good and some that are very destructive such as addiction, pride, and codependency. White fir brings these issues to the surface so that we can work through them and break destructive patterns.

Emotions: pride, jealousy, anger, arrogance, self-hatred, shame.

Affirmations: A river of compassion washes away my anger and replaces it with love. I cherish being able to stand out from the crowd. Through being myself, I form only healthy, lasting friendships. I release all the trauma, grief, and pain I am carrying in my mind, body, and energy field. I am grounded and secure.

Wild Orange *(Citrus sinensis)*. Wild orange is richly mood uplifting and encourages happiness, good health, and a lifetime of joy. It is a powerful essential oil to increase abundance in every area of life. Wild orange brings joy and rids the mind of fear and anxiety. It reminds the soul of innate, universal bliss. Combine wild orange with frankincense daily to support recovery from symptoms of depression. Use the two aromatically and topically for emotional clarity and daily joy.

Emotions: depression, grief, irritability, fear, self-criticism, trauma.

Affirmations: Creative energy surges through me and leads me to new and brilliant ideas. I release struggle and resistance. I am resilient and resourceful. I choose to see how every situation serves me.

Wintergreen *(Gaultheria fragrantissima).* Wintergreen is a natural painkiller. Physically, it can assist with headaches, joint pain, and tissue pain. It also relieves the emotional pain of those who inhale it. Wintergreen teaches us that we do not always need to be right. We can let go of the ways in which we hurt if we're carrying burdens of wrongdoing by others. It can help us release the pain associated with our own trials. It also teaches us that we do not need to carry burdens alone.

Emotions: anger, stress, aggravation, grief, guilt, overwhelm.

Affirmations: I am open to the possibility of peace. I feel centered in the peaceful loving energy of my heart. I can release my past and live calmly and serenely. No matter what events occur during the day, I remain calm and centered. I am open to receiving support. I bring peace into moments of chaos.

Ylang Ylang *(Cananga odorata).* Ylang Ylang helps us open our hearts and restore the child within us. It is physically useful for heart conditions. Ylang Ylang suggests to our minds and hearts that we can open to feel love, joy, and emotional safety. Consequently, ylang ylang can assist people who have gone through intense emotional traumas, helping them to let go of the pain and move forward in life.

Emotions: trauma, resistance, numbness, discouragement, fear.

Affirmations: I live bravely and boldly. I choose to see myself as whole and unbroken. My heart leads me to experience the best in life. Like the depths of the ocean, my mind is calm in each moment.

Essential Oil Blends

These oil blends are organized alphabetically by purpose.

Anti-aging blend (frankincense, sandalwood, lavender, myrrh). This blend of essential oils encourages spiritual well-being and growth. It encourages hope, faith, and gratitude while ridding the body and soul of consuming darkness. It helps us to be present in the moment and understand our spirits and the role of a divine power in our lives. Also, it's useful for the treatment of skin blemishes and wrinkles.

Calming blend (lavender, marjoram, Roman chamomile, ylang ylang). This blend of essential oils helps heal the heart and encourages us to forgive by reducing the impact on us of emotions such as hate, anger, fear, and resentment. As these emotions fade, we are able to feel more compassion for others and to accept that no one is perfect.

Cellular repair blend (frankincense, wild orange, lemongrass, thyme, summer savory). This blend repairs emotional patterns that are found in our DNA. It encourages individuals who feel they are stuck in those destructive patterns to see the light of a new day. It helps to shift the energy in the body and reminds us that we can change and life will get better. This blend works well for any mental health condition.

Cleansing blend (lemon, lime, pine, citronella). This powerful essential oil blend helps individuals who feel burdened by the toxicity of destructive habits and patterns. It cleanses the soul of heavy emotions, thereby providing space for emotional breakthroughs.

Comforting blend (frankincense, patchouli, ylang ylang, labdanum, amyris, sandalwood, rose, osmanthus). This blend helps soothe feelings of sadness and depression. If we are grieving the death of a loved one, it may ease the pain of our loss. It reminds us that we are whole in the part of us that is not bound to the body. The oils in this blend promote balance in the hormonal system, creating overall wellbeing.

Detoxification blend (clove, grapefruit, thyme, and geranium). This blend helps us cleanse our organs. It reduces the effect of harmful environment toxins and microbes that enter our bodies. Emotionally, it also aids us when we are going through changes and transitions.

Digestive blend (ginger, peppermint, tarragon, fennel, caraway). This blend is for those who struggle to digest the process of life, and thus, may feel overwhelmed and exhausted. It helps individuals see how to accomplish tasks one at a time, in a digestible fashion. It can cleanse the gut and by doing so, reestablish motivation by helping the brain receive peace and clearer instruction.

Encouraging blend (peppermint, clementine, coriander, basil, yuzu, Melissa, rosemary). In times of emotional uncertainty, this oil give us the courage we need to follow the path ahead of us. It reminds us of our own goodness and releases us from stress that comes from the negative belief that we "are not good enough." For those who are anxious about meeting a specific challenge, such as taking an important test or breaking bad news, it can calm the nerves and help with focus.

Feminine celebration blend (patchouli, bergamot, sandalwood, rose, jasmine, cinnamon, cistus, vetiver, ylang ylang). This blend celebrates feminine nature and supports female energy and body function. It helps to calm feelings of tension, reduce unhealthy pride and competitiveness, and can encourage positive nurturing and adaptability. It also can help a broken mother-child relationship. This blend is particularly helpful for helping women connect to their feminine side.

Focus blend (amyris, patchouli, frankincense, lime, ylang ylang). This blend is used to help individuals who have a hard time staying focus and finishing the task on hand. It is an excellent choice for those with ADHD symptoms or who work in a distracting environment, such as a shared office. The focus blend calms and grounds the mind, causing us to stay present in the moment and finish what is in front of us.

Grounding blend (spruce, ho wood, frankincense, blue tansy, blue chamomile). This blend is composed entirely of tree oils. Think of a tree rooting itself deep into the ground so it may grow tall and live long. Essential oils in the tree family remind us to be firmly rooted. When this blend is applied topically, it encourages us to reconnect to our roots and learn patience when trying to achieve goals. It teaches us to see the bigger perspective, find inner strength, and reestablish our lives in ways that help us grow tall and strong. This blend can help with jetlag, symptoms of depression, and headaches.

Headache relief blend. *(See Tension blend).*

Insect repellent blend (lemon, eucalyptus, citronella). This oil blend is a wonderful way to keep bugs away—including that which "bugs" us in life. Thus, it may serve as an emotional shield. Those who tend to hold others burdens and negative emotions will benefit from this blend. It helps us create emotionally boundaries so that we don't absorb and carry feelings that aren't ours.

Inspiring blend (cardamom, cinnamon, ginger, clove, sandalwood, jasmine, damiana). This powerful blend helps to restore our passion for life and helps instill us with the courage to pursue our dreams. It promotes enthusiasm and affection. Those who are working to achieve a great and important purpose will feel refreshed by its scent.

Invigorating blend (wild orange, lemon, grapefruit, mandarin, bergamot, tangerine). All citrus essential oils are natural mood lifters. They natural trigger a good mood, mental clarity, and feelings of peace and happiness. When blended together, these essential oils can support creativity of mind and a burst of joy, energy, and inner peace. Everyone has the right to create. This blend helps us imagine and have confidence in our creations. Through using the creative part of the brain, we then feel the spark of life again. This blend can encourage happiness when diffused and is an excellent daily blend to diffuse at home or at the office.

Joyful blend (lavandin, tangerine, elemi, lemon myrtle, Melissa, ylang ylang). This blend is for individuals who are depressed. It cleanses energy and calms the heart. It makes the heart more open to relaxation, joy, courage, and light by encouraging us to reach our goals. It may teach us that fear and worry don't need to take us down and we can get what we want in life. This blend is particularly helpful for emotional imbalance that may surface with symptoms of depression.

Massage blend (basil, grapefruit, cypress, marjoram). This blend is used to help the mind and body relax. It helps ease tension in the body. It also helps to soothe the souls of people who are going through sorrow or feel overwhelmed with stress. By helping them relax and let go on a deep level, energy can start freely moving again through their bodies. This helps people move forward in life peacefully.

Metabolic blend (grapefruit, lemon, peppermint, and ginger). This essential oil is for individuals who struggle with loving their bodies. It encourages self-worth and helps release negative emotions about body image. It seeks to regulate metabolism, and in doing so, may regulate emotions that prevent healthy digestion of the life's natural ebbs and flows. As we work through issues related to body image and metabolizing life, we may learn to love our and honor our human body and appreciate the miracle and blessing that it is for us.

Protective blend (wild orange, clove, cinnamon). This blend helps strengthen the immunity and provides us with physical protection from viruses and harmful bacteria. Emotionally, this blend protects us by strengthening our inner selves, encouraging us to stand up for what we believe. It helps us to create boundaries and not let harmful energy around us into our personal energy field where it may deplete us.

Reassuring blend (vetiver, lavender, ylang ylang, frankincense, clary sage, marjoram, labdanum, spearmint). This blend is appropriate for times of worry when negative thoughts are swirling in the mind and we just can't let them go. Those who tend to obsess about their plans for the future at the expense of being present in the now may find this blend helps them to relax and find more contentment in the moment.

Renewing blend (spruce, bergamot, juniper berry, myrrh, arborvitae, nootka tree, thyme, citronella). If we are troubled by past decisions or feel guilty and ashamed about our choices or actions, this blend can help us forgive ourselves and find resolution. It takes weight off the mind and soothes the heart. Renewal of the spirit often comes during moments of prayer, meditation, or contemplation—and this oil blend enhances those experiences elevating and grounding simultaneously.

Respiratory blend (laurel leaf, peppermint, eucalyptus, melaleuca). This oil blend supports a healthy life through breathing and releasing grief and pain that may be taking the breath right out of us. As we take a breath in and out each day, we have the opportunity to let go and allow new life and possibilities to enter our mind and body. This blend encourages us to do just that--to balance our life by breathing out what hurts and breathing in encouragement, light, and hope for a restful and joyful future. Physically, this blend is helpful for respiratory issues and can support healthy breathing.

Restful blend (lavender, cedarwood, ho wood, ylang ylang, marjoram, Roman chamomile, vetiver, Hawaiian sandalwood). This blend addresses the emotional states that can interfere with sleep. Whether it is stress, excitement, or anxiety that keeps us from letting go of the day or staying asleep in the middle of the night, this oil blend is a companion we can trust to help us feel calmer so we may rest.

Skin-clearing blend (black cumin seed, rosewood, melaleuca, eucalyptus). This blend has very positive properties that help with skin health. Emotionally, it helps individuals that have suppressed emotions (such as anger and guilt) reduce a tendency to lash out at people. This blend encourages self-acceptance and healthy release of negative emotions. It's particularly helpful for relieving feelings of aggravation, self-hate, or self-rejection that may surface through the skin as acne.

Soothing blend (wintergreen, camphor, peppermint, blue tansy, blue chamomile). This blend helps release emotional issues that may be causing physical pain. By bringing struggle and agony to the surface, it can be released and consequently, may relieve the physical body of pain and trauma. Consequently, this blend is helpful for physical pain management.

Tension blend (wintergreen, lavender, peppermint, frankincense, cilantro, Roman chamomile, marjoram). Also known as the headache relief blend, this blend helps individuals who are emotionally overwhelmed to let go of the stress that may be causing tension in the body. It helps to calm and relax the mind so that tension can be resolved and released. This blend is particularly helpful for treatment of headaches and migraines associated with fear, anger, frustration, resentment, and other forms of emotional upset.

Uplifting blend (wild orange, clove, star anise, lemon myrtle, nutmeg, cinnamon). When we need to cheer up or promote positivity in a particular environment, this may be the blend of choice. Highly distressed people may find that it helps heal their hearts. Those who are down in the dumps or just feel sluggish and disengaged may find that it spices things up for them and restores their enthusiasm for living.

Women's monthly blend (clary sage, lavender, bergamot, Roman chamomile, cedarwood, ylang ylang, geranium, fennel, carrot seed). This essential oil blend supports healthy relationships. It teaches us to be open and vulnerable at times so that we may rid ourselves of the fear of rejection. It helps us maintain emotional balance within our life by teaching us to safely accept the ideas, thoughts, and feelings of others who love us. In turn, it helps us to feel love in our relationships. It's useful for addressing emotions related to women's monthly cycles.

References

American Psychological Association (APA). (2006). "Forgiveness: A Sampling of Research Results." Washington, D.C.: Office of International Affairs.

Blumenthal, J. A., et al. (2007). "Exercise and pharmacotherapy in the treatment of major depressive disorder." Psychosom Med 69(7):587–96.

Braden, Gregg. (2006). *The Divine Matrix: Bridging Time, Space, Miracles, and Belief.* San Francisco: Hay House.

Burr, W. R., et al. (2012). *Sacred Matters: Religion and Spirituality in Families.* New York: Routledge.

Cappello, G., et al.(2007). "Peppermint oil in the treatment of irritable bowel syndrome: a prospective double blind placebo controlled randomized trial." Digestive Liver Dis 39(6):530–6.

Chopra, Deepak (1994). *The Seven Spiritual Laws of Success.* San Rafael, CA: Amber-Allen Publishing.

Covey, Stephen R. (1982). *The Divine Center.* Salt Lake City, UT: Book-craft.

Dalai Lama. (1989). Nobel Lecture. http://www.nobelprize.org/ nobel_prizes/peace/laureates/1989/lama-lecture.html. Last accessed August 2012.

Dew, S. L. (2003). "You were born to lead, you were born for glory." 2003–2004 Speeches. Provo, UT.: Brigham Young University Press.

Friedman, M., et al. (2002). "Bactericidal activities of plant essential oils and some of the isolated constituents against Campylobacter jejuni, Escherichia coli, listeria monocytogenes, and Salmonella enterica." J Food Prot. 65(10):1545–60.

Fuchs, S. M., et al.(2005). "Protective effects of different marigold (Calenddula officinalas L.) and rosemary cream preparations against sodium-lauryl-sulfate-induced irritant contact dermatitis." Skin Pharmacol Physiol 18(4):195–200.

Griebel, V. (2008). "The power of intention." http://www.drwaynedyer.com/articles/the-power-of-intention. Last accessed August 2012.

Hafen, B.Q., et al. (1992). "The Health Effects of Attitudes, Emotions, Relationships." Provo, UT.: EMS Associates.

Hendrix, H. (1998). *Getting the Love You Want: A Guide for Couples.* New York: Henry Holt and Company.

Hintze, R. L. (2006). *Healing Your Family History: 5 Steps to Break Free of Destructive Patterns.* San Francisco: Hay House.

Kahn, A., et al. (2003). "Cinnamon improves glucose and lipids of people with type 2 diabetes." Diabetes Care 26(12): 3215–18.

Keller, H. (2004). *The Story of My Life: The Restored Edition.* New York: Random House.

Lipton, B. H. (2008). *The Biology of Belief: Unleashing the Power of Consciousness, Matter, & Miracles.* Hay House.

Lucado, M. (2002). *If Only I Had a Green Nose.* Wheaton, IL.: Crossway.

Maharaj, M. and Kathrada, A., eds. (2006). *Mandela: The Authorized Portrait.* Kansas City, MO.: Andrews McMeel.

Mayer, R. (2007). "Purification of citrus limonoids and their differential inhibitory effects on human cytochrome P450 enzymes." Journal of Science of Food and Agriculture 87:1699–1709

McCullough, L.E., et al. (2012). "Fat or fit: The joint effects of physical activity, weight gain, and body size on breast cancer risk." Cancer.

Mehrabian, A. (1972). *Nonverbal Communication.* Chicago, IL.: Aldine-Atherton.

Montgomery, L.M. (1990). *Anne of Avonlea.* Illustrated Junior Library. New York: Grosset & Dunlap.

NAMI.   (2009).   Major   Depression   Fact   Sheet. http://www.nami.org/Template.cfm?Section=Depression&Template=/ContentManagement/ContentDisplay.cfm&ContentID=88956. Last accessed August 2012.

NIH.   (2007).   Brain   Basics: Understanding   Sleep. http://www.ninds.nih.gov/disorders/brain_basics/understanding_sleep.htm. Last accessed August 2012.

Orstein, R. and Sobel, D. (1990). *The Healing Brain: a Scientific Reader.* New York: The Guilford Press, p. 88.

Pattnaik, S., et al. (1996). "Antibacterial and antifungal activity of ten essential oils in vitro." Microbios. 86(349):237–46.

Pert, C. (1995). Neuropeptides, AIDS and the science of mind-body healing. Alternative Therapies in Health and Medicine. 1(3):70-76.

———. (1997). Molecules of Emotion: Why You Feel the Way You Feel. New York: Scribner.

Salovey, P. andMayer, J. D. (1990). "Emotional intelligence." Imagination, Cognition, and Personality. 9:185–211.

Sarrell, E. M., et al.. (2003). "Naturopathic treatment for ear pain in children." Pediatrics 111:e574–9.

Schiller, F. (1871). *The Poems of Schiller, Complete.* Henry D. Wireman, tran. Philadelphia: I. Kohler.

Stevens, N. (2009). *Essential Oil Cancer Research*. Brochure. Abundant Health.

Taylor, Eldon (2007). *Choices and Illusions: How Did I Get Where I Am, and How Do I Get Where I Want to Be?* San Francisco: Hay House.

Valnet, Jean. (1980). *The Practice of Aroma Therapy: A Classic Compendium of Plant Medicines and Their Healing Properties*. Edited by Robert Tisserand. Rochester, VT.: Healing Arts Press.

Van Oyen Witvliet, C., et al. (2001). "Granting forgiveness or harboring grudges: implications for emotion, physiology, and health." Psychological Science. 2, 117–23.

———. (2000) Zest magazine.

Wansink, B. and Chandon, P. (2006). Can "low-fat" nutrition labels lead to obesity? Journal of Marketing Research. 43(4), 605–17.

Williamson, Marianne (2006). *A Return to Love.* New York: Harper Paperbacks.

Acknowledgments

I am most grateful to my husband, Shane Hintze, for his belief in me and his support. I am also grateful to my children, Ashley Hintze Beans, Nicholas Hintze, Kathryn Hintze, and Michael Hintze. These amazing individuals have provided me with my greatest joy in life.

I would like to thank my son Nick for supplying an excellent cover for this book, and my assistant Melissa McCafferty for her support.

I am deeply thankful for the editorial skills of Janna DeVore and Stephanie Gunning, who helped make the book read well.

ABOUT THE AUTHOR

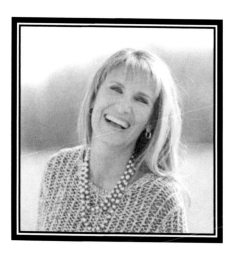

Rebecca Linder Hintze, M.Sc., is a family issues expert, former broadcast journalist, and bestselling author of *Healing Your Family History* (Hay House, 2006), which has been translated into eight languages, and *Essentially Happy* (Visium Books, 2014). She holds a bachelor's degree from Brigham Young University and a master of science degree from University of East London, School of Psychology. A mother of four grown children, she currently resides in Northern Virginia with her husband, Shane.